AMISH

FOLK REMEDIES

For Plain and Fancy Ailments

by William R. McGrath

ISBN. 0-9617405-8-2

This book is a collection of historic Amish folk remedies. The reporting herein of any remedy is not a claim for its curative powers nor a guarantee of its effectiveness. This information is not for diagnosing nor prescribing. The author and publisher assume no responsibility for anyone who uses this information. It is not the purpose of this book to replace the services of a physician. Use your common sense and see your doctor for any condition requiring his help.

Publishers retail price $6.99
"Amish Folk Remedies" available at bookstores
or contact:

S. Chupp's Books
27539 Londick
Burr Oak, Mich. 49030

First Printing	Dec. 1984
Second Printing	Feb. 1985
Third Printing	July 1985 (Revised Edition)
Fourth Printing	Oct. 1986
Fifth Printing	Oct. 1988
Sixth Printing	June 1993

Table of Contents

Preface:

The Value of Folk Medicine. Here are some views of folk medicine, written by medical doctors:

"Through their long history, the Amish have been a sturdy people who have withstood persecution and economic depression. Having large families and low income, they are often slow (sometimes too slow) to come to a physician for help in time of illness or accident. They have tried the simple materials at home, sometimes without success; but when these do succeed, they can be eminently useful in alleviating common ailments. They are not cure-alls, however, and no substitute for a physician when illness is serious. We are glad for this collection of the home remedies [often natural], that have succeeded, written by a scholarly and qualified author, and highly recommend it for your reading."

—G. Richard Culp, D. O.

Dr. Andrew Weil, M.D., research associate of the Harvard Botanical Museum, and a practicing physician, says: "I believe very strongly that a plant in its natural form is different from a chemical substance that has been isolated and purified. Medicinal plants are complex mixtures of things. One chemical may be principally responsible for its activity, but secondary components modify the effect—they aren't just inert. [But] a refined drug goes into the bloodstream faster, *with a greater risk of toxicity.* There's an interaction of all the components of the natural preparation that makes it safer and more effective." (—Dr. Weil himself instructs his patients to drink ephedra leaf tea instead of prescribing ephedrine drugs!)

Dr. Halfdan Mahler, Director General of the World Health Organization wrote: "The age-old arts of the herbalists must be tapped. Many of the plants familiar to the wise woman...really do have the healing powers that tradition attaches to them."

5

Dr. James A. Duke, chief of the Department of Agriculture's Economic Botany Laboratory, writes: "The search for agents to fight cancer, that's our main thrust right now. We're likely to find twice as many effective agents among folk remedies as among random samples." There is even a new interest in folk therapies that have nothing to do with drugs.

Dr. Andrew Weil says: "The old folk customs for treating sickness are worth following. Get a lot of rest, drink fluids, eat less. I agree with tradition on the value of sweating. I tell my patients to take saunas or drink hot liquids [teas]. These simple remedies for sickness are often just a way of following our instincts. But it's amazing how many people don't follow them. Rather than going to bed and resting—they take a pill!"

European studies have proven that *garlic* contains an antibiotic called allicin. Even in the U.S., Dr. Moses Attrep Jr., of East Texas State University, investigating onions and garlic by gas chromatography-mass spectometry, confirmed the presence of prostaglandin A-1, a hormone-like substance that can *lower blood pressure!* But despite such evidences, the average medical doctor keeps on making such statements:

Folk Medicine Lacking Proper Antibiotics! by Dr. R.B. (MD). Q. *My husband's infected foot was cured by an old neighbor lady who wrapped it in tansy leaves. Why?* A. Folk medicine may have values we don't understand but you might lose a limb without using proper antibiotics! Tansy oil is said to be poisonous, so be careful.
Q. *My 90-year-old grandmother takes lots of garlic, saying it keeps blood pressure down and promotes long life. Is that true?* A. There is no experimental evidence that I know of."

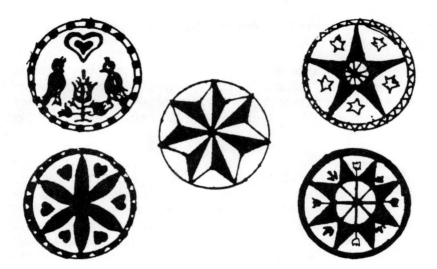

Chapter 1: **Amish Folk Remedies and Health Recipes**

Shown above are 5 common Pennsylvania Dutch symbols. They are *not* "hex signs" but folk art symbols of man's striving for happiness through harmony with God and nature. The 5-pointed star of Saul, 6-pointed star of David, 7-pointed star of Bethlehem, 8-pointed star of the New Covenant, all symbolize submission to God's rule.

The tulips symbolize the Trinity, the Rose and the Lily refer to Christ, the hearts to being open to God's love, and the doves to peace and the Holy Spirit. All these symbols point to the Amish belief that health and happiness is found in harmony between God, man and nature.

In the modern world where urban man has polluted his environment and is armed to the teeth against his fellow man, the Amish survive as a reminder of a peaceful, rural folk culture. They have survived for centuries by pursuing simplicity and quietness, instead of wealth and power. They have also preserved health recipes to share with anybody listening.

It is typical of our modern cynicism to misinterpret such symbols as "hex signs." Long before they ever appeared on barns, such symbols were put on Pennsylvania Dutch furniture, quilts, plates, and even Bible covers. If anyone is "hexed," it is our arrogant commentators who dismiss all folk cultures as "primitive" if they have chosen a less frantic lifestyle.

The purpose of this book is to introduce you to the practical home remedies of a pioneer people who survive in our midst but are unknown. The Amish are pioneer survivors of a more self-sufficient time. They can teach us practical survival skills even in the midst of our urban jungle, where medical costs have shot sky-high.

We do not expect that our readers will all want to join the Amish! However, it would be wise for all of us to become acquainted with survival skills in these troubled times. We are not advocating that you give up doctors and hospitals, but just that you have a handy survival manual full of *first aid* hints that anybody can use. All of the ingredients of these recipes can be found in your local health food store. If you are a camper or hiker, you will be able to find many of them in nature. They are much cheaper than prescription drugs, and undoubtedly have fewer side-effects!

Understanding the Biblical Background: The Amish health views are based on the Biblical background of both the Old and New Testaments. The Bible itself claims that Moses was learned in all the wisdom of the Egyptians. His inspired sanitary regulations were unsurpassed until modern times. One of the main writers of the New Testament was Luke, a "beloved physician" trained in the best Greek and Roman therapies. Nowadays there has been a return to the **wholistic** approach of the Biblical world-view. Man **is** to be healthy in **body, soul, and spirit.**

The health ideal of classical times was "a sound mind in a sound body." This is also the Biblical view. Surprisingly modern, even futuristic standards of health and happiness are taught in the Bible. The Amish try to incorporate these Biblical ideals in their own lifestyle.

For example, in the Old Testament book of *Proverbs*, there is outlined a divine plan for a society in which people work hard, respect each other's rights, treat the less fortunate kindly, are concerned for the welfare of the poor, and seek to maintain a general atmosphere of friendliness. They are supposed to enjoy the pleasures of moderation, love their families and homes, be sincere, modest, self-controlled, temperate, reliable, pure, willing to listen and learn, forgiving, considerate, discreet, kind to animals, liberal givers, and yet prudent and providing for their own families. This is also the Amish ideal, by which they try to live.

Furthermore, the Amish seek to reproduce that further New Testament ideal of being peacemakers in the midst of a cut-throat world of competition and arms races. They deliberately opted to deny themselves some modern gadgets (automobiles, electricity, expensive machinery, television, and the latest Paris fashions), in order to concentrate more on basic humanity. Their ideal is expressed in these New Testament words: "God hath not given us the spirit of fear; but of power, and of love, and of a sound mind." (II Tim. 1:7). They call this **the mind and the Spirit of Christ,** and seek to live it by God's grace.

So much for the theological basis of the Amish lifestyle. What anybody can profit from are many of their remarkable health recipes. For example, even in their farming, their goal is not to merely raise better crops and livestock, but to **raise better people,** with a more humane system of mutual aid.

Classifying Amish health therapies: You would not expect the average Amishman to be able to explain what we are going to say next. They do these things by tradition and common sense, rather than conscious planning. Since I am both an Amish-Mennonite minister and a trained natural therapist, I shall be able to explain the system to you in such a way that you will be able to choose for yourself many practical first aid techniques.

Examine the following diagram. It shows seven basic therapies or areas of health practices followed by the Amish. All seven together comprise a harmonious system of health that could be followed by anybody who wished to adopt it.

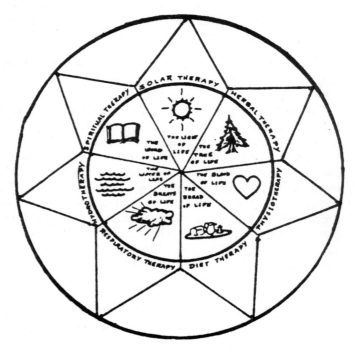

A *therapy* is simply one area of health practices. You can see from the table of contents how these 7 classifications work, so that you may find the answer to many health questions.

Explanation of the therapy systems:

1. Solar Therapy refers to the healing power of light energy (the light of life). All of our foods are really derived from sunlight energy mediated to us through plants and animals. So here we group health questions relating to our **immuno-defensive** system, and discuss energy and fatigue, vitamins and minerals, strength and debility, infections, fevers, headaches, parasites that can sap our strength, colors, sleep.

2. Herbal Therapy refers to the healing power in herbs, especially in relation to the body's **reproductive system** (the tree of life). Problems relating to sex, pregnancy, potency, menopause, etc. are discussed.

3. Physiotherapy relates to health problems of the **circulatory and skeleto-muscular system** (The Blood of life): heart, arteries, circulation, blood pressure, muscle aches, joints, bones, etc.

4. Diet Therapy refers to problems of the **digestive system** (the bread of life). This includes balanced diet, indigestion, obesity, fasting, etc.

5. Respiratory Therapy (the breath of life). Here we include for convenience the nose, throat, eyes and ears, sinus, lungs, all together under the **respiratory system**.

6. Hydrotherapy relates to problems of the **skin and eliminatory system** (keeping clean through the water of life). The skin is the body's largest organ of elimination and we study its problems as well as hair, nails, kidneys, bowels, burns, fungus, poisons, acne, etc.

7. Spiritual Therapy is the 7th category (the Word of life) and relates to problems of the **nervous system** and personality. Here we look at remedies for fear, depression, nervousness, etc.

All of these categories are interrelated, of course. If you do not know where to look up the answer to a certain health problem, just use the cross index at the back of the book · where ailments are listed alphabetically.

First Aid: Remember that the purpose of this book is to help you find quick answers to minor health problems. Reporting as we do in this book the home remedies of the Amish is in no way any guarantee of cures or encouragement for you to bypass your family doctor when some chronic or grave problem requires his professional expertise. As with any survival manual, you use it best with common sense!

'For example, suppose your boy was stung by a wasp. This happened to our ten year old son, some years ago. He got such a quantity of venom that he went into anaphylactic shock and almost died. We had to take him to the emergency room of a nearby hospital for an injection. The doctor there assured us that he would have to ever afterwards carry cortisone tablets at all times or be in mortal danger. *Since then we learned that a raw onion applied at once to the site of the sting will effectively remove the venom, stop the swelling, and anesthetize the pain!* You cut the onion in half and simply hold the dripping half pressed over the sting until the pain is gone.

There are dozens of simple first aid measures like this that could save your life or avoid much expense and unpleasantness. Most of the ingredients for these Amish remedies are available at your local health food store, grocery store or drug store. Simple directions are given for their use.

The Plain People and Health Remedies: Ever since the Anabaptists of Reformation times (1525 and following), Plain People have applied themselves to discovering simple health remedies. The Anabaptist Mennonites not only tried to return to New Testament Christianity, they also restudied classical Greek and Roman health remedies. They practiced d'et and fasting, baths and massage, exercise, rest, and herbalism. Early Hutterite Anabaptists became famous for their health spas in which massage, bonesetting, hot baths and herbs were used for the sick.

In 1750, Hans Plank, an Amish Mennonite herb doctor and minister, fled from Switzerland to escape persecution. After two years in Germany, he came to Pennsylvania in 1752. There he practiced his Amish faith and his profession of herbalism. Some of the recipes we give in this book are from his direct descendants who are still practicing Amish herbalists!

The first real medicinal herb garden in America is said to have been the botanic plantings of Quaker John Bartram, who searched the whole colony for native plants and trees to begin his garden in Philadelphia by 1728.

Later the Shakers developed one of the first American herb businesses, growing, collecting, drying and processing hundreds of thousands of dollars worth of herbal medicines in the 1800's. Their single herbs, salves, tinctures, and herbal compounds were famous for potency and quality. They were also the first Americans to package seeds and sell them.

Even today, the Amish are involved in the herb business. The Amish family newspaper, called *The Sugarcreek Budget* (a weekly paper from Sugarcreek, Ohio 44681), contains many advertisements for those in the herb business. In its columns you may read of not only traditional American and European herbs for sale, but also of exotic Oriental herbs, as well as the latest jungle herbs imported from Brazil and Paraguay!

A Shaker elder wrote in 1875: "I hold that no man who lives as we do has a right to be ill before he is sixty." Another advocate of the simple life, Henry David Thoreau, wrote: "A man may esteem himself happy when that which is his food is also his medicine." An anonymous Amish poet wrote in 1974:

OLD TIME REMEDIES

I sort of want to give a list
O' Mother's famous cures;
There'll be, of course, some that she missed
Which may be found in yours.

In spring we took our sassafras,
Molasses-sulphur mix,
To clean our blood, make us first class
When we got out of fix.

Her catnip and her boneset tea
Were taken 'stead of pills;
We didn't dare refuse this need
For curin' all our ills.

By rubbing goose grease on our chest
She'd cure most any cold
While mustard, lamp-oil 'n the rest
Might also be extolled.

Her poultices were mighty fine
O' flaxseed 'n o' bread,
'N fat-meat, onions, this whole line
Would bring things to a head.

But strikes me it was Mother love
That really made us well,
A healin' sent from heaven above
That worked her magic spell.

For when she'd tuck us snug in bed
And give that tender kiss,
Ain't nothing further need be said
'Bout such a cure as this!

I had the pleasure of curing myself of crippling rheumatoid arthritis, and also of asthma. No wonder Ecclesiasticus 38:4 (Apocrypha) says: "The Lord hath created medicines out of the earth!"

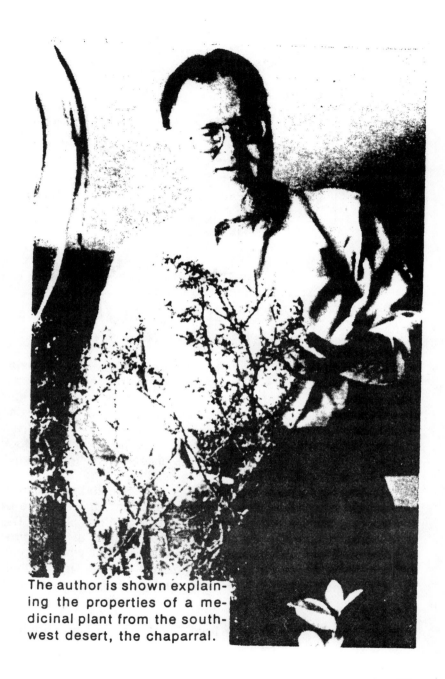

The author is shown explaining the properties of a medicinal plant from the southwest desert, the chaparral.

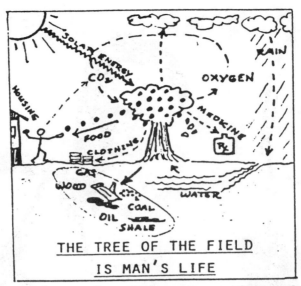

THE TREE OF THE FIELD
IS MAN'S LIFE

Chapter 2: **Recipes for the Immuno-Defensive System**

The Bible says, *"The tree of the field is man's life."* (Deut. 20:19). This refers to mankind's dependence on the plant kingdom. It is plants that take the radiant energy of the light of the sun and transform it into organic energy which we can eat and absorb. 60 to 67% of our diet comes directly from plants and the other 33 to 40% comes from livestock indirectly fed by plants. Eating plants, we eat **light**-energy!

In 1936, Dr. Bircher-Benner of Switzerland stated: "Absorption and organization of *sunlight*, the essence of life, takes place almost exclusively within plants. The organs of the plant are, therefore, a kind of *biological accumulation of light*. They are the basis of what we call food, whence animal and human bodies derive their substance and energy. Hence, **sunlight** is the driving force of the cells of our body."

God said, "Let there be **light**!" Light energy is our life. But

16

many today are eating artificially preserved foods with little *light energy*!

It is a fact that people were designed to eat fresh foods. When we eat too many stale foods (preserved and processed), we lose many of the light energy vitamins and enzymes we need. Our domesticated food crops, mass-produced and forced by chemical fertilizers, do not have the *light energy* found in more natural foods.

So our first principle of health in this chapter will be to maintain that *fresh foods* supply us with more *light energy* to equip our immuno-defensive system against the invasion of disease. All of us are living all the time in a sea of bacteria. Some of us are better able to withstand these invaders because our bodies have the fresh enzymes and vitamins and light energy we need!

An Amish family works outside as much as possible in the fresh air and sunshine. As much of their food as possible is taken from their own gardens and orchards. An Amish man told me once of how he was different from European neighbors who had emigrated to where he was living in Paraguay. They complained that the cost of beer and soda pop was too high! He laughed and said, "We drink *water*, you know!" Pure food and pure water energize our immuno-defensive system against many of the degenerative diseases so common in modern society.

Our average American diet, according to the 1977 Senate report on nutrition, is capable of killing **6 out of 10 Americans dying from the major diseases:** heart trouble, cancer, diabetes, strokes, arteriosclerosis, overweight, cirrhosis of the liver, and respiratory disease. This comes from too much fat, sugar, salt, alcohol, refined flour, starch, preserved meats!

Study the two food charts on the next page. The one has a low light energy content and breeds disease. The other defends you!

Which Diet Has More Light Energy for Health?

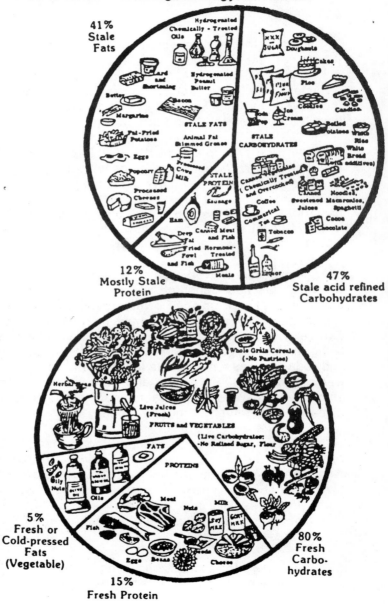

41%
Stale
Fats

12%
Mostly Stale
Protein

47%
Stale acid refined
Carbohydrates

5%
Fresh or
Cold-pressed
Fats
(Vegetable)

15%
Fresh Protein

80%
Fresh
Carbo-
hydrates

So eat fresh foods and drink pure water and juices! But you will say, how can we do that in the city? Establish a miniature farm on your kitchen sink! Get untreated seeds of alfalfa, mung beans, sunflower, lentils, radish, wheat grass, rye, corn, rice, peas and millet. Soak them overnight; pour them onto a sprouting tray; rinse them 3 to 5 times daily to prevent souring; keep them covered with a warm, wet cloth. Eat when they are 3 to 5 days old. The sprouted seeds *increase* in vitamins, minerals, enzymes, amino acids and sunlight **energy** from 30 to 600% over the dry seeds! Start an Amish kitchen-garden today!

For pure water, get yourself a juicer and juice organically grown fruits and vegetables. Get a water distiller or water filter (reverse osmosis type) and take noxious chemicals out of your water. For fresher air, move out into the country, even if you take a cut in salary! Or fill your apartment with growing plants, because they feed on your exhaled carbon dioxide and in turn they increase the *oxygen* in the air!

Remember that herbs are often collected from the wild, and have more light energy than mass produced crops. Drink plenty of herbal teas, instead of black tea, coffee, or soda pop (which have too many chemicals such as tannin, caffeine, sugar, and dyes). Powerful cancer-causing cleaning fluids are used in decaffeinating coffee and a residue can remain in it!

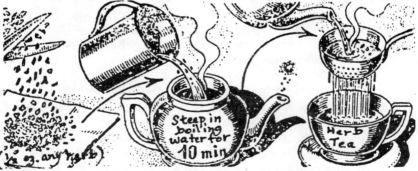

Any bark tea: slowly boil ten minutes. Then steep ten minutes.

Sun tea? Some enjoy making "sun tea." You take any fresh herbs (or dried) and place them in a glass gallon jar or jug, cap it tightly after filling it with fresh or mineral water, and then place it to bake and steep for hours in the direct sunlight. Sweeten with honey to taste.

Remedies for disordered immuno-defense system: So far, we have considered *preventives,* which are the best remedy. Now let's examine some old Amish recipes. First, let's consider *tonics.* These are designed to invigorate, strengthen or tone up a debilitated system. Here is a recipe from a naturopathic doctor who had been raised Amish:

"My grandmother used to use what she called Snake Root bark, boiled down into a syrup, mixed with honey. This was used as a *spring tonic* [to produce perspiration, make for a keener appetite, and tranquilize a nervous stomach]." The medicinal name is Aristolochia serpentaria, and it is used today in drug form as a tranquilizer, also for high blood pressure. A half ounce of the dried root may be steeped in a pint of boiling water for 2 hours, before taking by the teaspoonful, 3 times daily. [Mint tea with rue is another fine tonic.]

Watercress leaves, with their high sulphur content, are a good spring *tonic*; eat as a salad. Dandelion leaves make a vitamin-rich tonic salad. Alfalfa sprouts are a good tonic. Also, a good home-made ginger ale can be made by chopping up a ginger root, simmering until water is dark yellow (1 quart), straining, and adding honey and carbonated mineral water.

Dandelion wine is a spring *tonic* made by soaking 3 quarts of the flowers in 2 quarts of water for 72 hours; strain, add 2 lbs. sugar, 1 sliced lemon, 1 tblsp. yeast; let it stand for 96 hours, then bottle it. Use 1 tblsp. before meals, as needed. Another good tonic is a homemade root beer. One of the main ingredients, sarsaparilla, is a good hormone stimulant. Take 2 oz. each of sarsaparilla root, sassafras root, spikenard root, black birch bark, yellow dock root, and spruce needles. Boil all of these together in 4 gallons of water for 25 minutes; strain; when cool add 1 pound brown sugar, and 3 tblsp. yeast. Let it ferment (make vent for escape of gas). Bottle after 3 days.

Tea made from Stinging Nettles boiled with honey added, is a good spring tonic. It is very high in vitamin and mineral content. But handle it with gloves! It also has been known to be a good tea for backaches.

Use of light and color: your body can be made sick by looking through the wrong color glasses; avoid any shade of red. If you must have a tinted lens, blue or green is the safest. Sick animals have been cured by just placing them under blue skylights! Never look at ultraviolet lights, it is harmful to the eyes. If you have florescent bulbs, use only the full daylight spectrum.

Psychologically, red agitates; families with red carpets have had many quarrels! Blue rugs and walls are calming for a bedroom. Green, blue or tan walls are conducive to meditation, and thus ideal for a church building.

The master gland of the body, the pituitary gland, regulates many body processes and is itself affected by the kind of light your eyes get. Many Amish use color lamps for light treatments of ailing limbs. Medical science recognizes the effect of infra-red and ultraviolet but is skeptical about the rest. Experiments have shown that light therapy can cure irregular menstrual cycles. Intensity and duration of light affects many body glands. For this reason it is important to have natural sunlight daily.

Caution should be exercised to avoid baking your skin in too much intense sunlight. This not only roughens the skin but can cause skin cancers. Amish men usually wear hats and the women wear bonnets. While Amish wear plain colors (not checked or striped but solid one color), they do like pastel colored shirts and dresses in shades of blue, blue-green, green and lavender. They love colorful gardens but shun artificial flowers. By the way, fresh flowers buried in dry sand for two weeks will become permanently preserved and may be made into attractive bouquets to last all year long.

Vitamins and minerals: Amish children in Pennsylvania eat the wild violets, which are higher in vitamin C than rose hips (and are also a traditional cancer preventive). Children who have contact with nature are more likely to absorb the vital nutrients they need than city children who lead sterile lives. One five year old boy, pale and anemic, listless and without energy, was cured by simply placing him to play day after day in a sand box!

One of the ancient remedies, for *debility* and removing body poisons, was the Greek therapy of mud baths in volcanic mud, hot springs waters, and/or immersion by the sea shore in wet sand for hours at a time. The body is thus ennabled to eliminate its toxins and absorb missing minerals!

Edible clay provides mineral treatments in some countries. Amish also use the kao lin Chinese clay to treat diarrhea (available as kao pectate). Clay masques are used to purify the facial pores. Clay poultices are used on stubborn sores. (Ancients even used clay poultice to put on sore eyes.) One way or another, a healthy person will absorb his quota of dirt!

One thing to beware of, in dirt contaminated by pet animals like cats and dogs, worm eggs can be present.

The Amish love animals and are very kind to them. But health-conscious Amish families realize that many different kinds of *parasites* can be caught from animals kept in the house (cats, dogs, birds). So the animals' place is outside. We know of cases where this was not done and unfortunate health problems arose. Birds such as parrots and parakeets can transmit a microorganism called Chlamydia psittaci, which leads to valvular heart damage and death. Turtles can transmit salmonella. Many a small child has suffered miserably from *fevers* caused by cat scratches, dog heart worms, etc.

Vitamins are basically biocatalysts, coenzymes and detoxifiers. They help all the body processes to work better. Vitamin A is known as the anti-infective vitamin and is found in fish liver oils, eggs, and liver. Vitamin B1 deficiency may lead to *weakness, mental depression and general lassitude.* The best sources are in brown rice, oat meal, and whole wheat, unless one takes a B complex capsule. General lassitude, dizziness, nervousness, are often seen in B-deficient children. Liver, yeast, fish oils, eggs and fresh milk are the antidote.

Vitamin C in 1000 milligram dosages is a good adult reinforcement, but may cause kidney irritation in small children. Amish often buy citrus fruit by the case in the winter, to supply their families. There is another favorite Amish *remedy for debility and lack of appetite* accompanied by thin hair and constant *sore throats.* They use red clover tops tea (or liquid tincture of red clover tops). This is packed so full of vitamins and minerals that it has made dramatic changes in *underweight, thin-haired,* sick' children. (It is also available in health food stores.) The clover, like the alfalfa, is a powerful concentrate of minerals for body defenses.

Besides fresh milk from the farm, many Amish use *calcium supplements* (bone meal, for example). Those familiar with herbs know which to take that are rich in the various minerals: lambs' quarters and okra pods for calcium; watercress for chlorine, sulphur; dandelion and nettle for iron; kelp for iodine; mullein leaves for magnesium; garlic for phosphorus; red grape juice for potassium; oatstraw for silicon; red clover tops for everything!

Many cases of weakened resistance to disease are due to *parasites.* Male fern root is an antidote to many kinds of worms, as is also garlic. An Amish family in Belize told me of a neighbor cured from cancer of the esophagus by drinking a tea made of fern root.

A favorite Amish home remedy for **weakness** is the use of ginseng root, chewed slowly all day long. Like garlic, ginseng is one of the herbs which emits mitogenetic radiation. Amish children and men hunt the ginseng roots in the woods, in order to resell them. Ginseng helps one meet **stress**. Another herb being used among the Amish is guarana, a Paraguayan stimulant to keep one awake. They also take a couple B-15 tablets from health stores for extra pep.

Alfalfa leaf tea is drunk to cure **undulant fever.** Elder blossom tea is good for bringing down *fever* in children. Yarrow tea has restored more than one sickly person to health again. One Amish girl was bothered with recurrent **high fevers**, until her parents found that one egg white beat with a fork, in one-sixth cup of cold water would bring the fever down. Strawberry leaf tea is for fever, too.

Fatigue: Tansy tea is an old Amish remedy for this. An afternoon nap of a half hour is equal to two hours of sleep at night. Another good **energizer** is chia seed; soak it overnight and drink in the morning a glass with one tablespoonful of the seeds. Lobelia tea is very good for breaking a *fever* (½ tsp./cup).

Poisons: A word should be said here about poisons. Two of the herbs just mentioned, tansy and lobelia, are regarded as poisons by the U.S. government. However, the quantity used in a cup of tea (less than 1 tsp. of dried herb or 5 to 10 drops of liquid tincture) is so small it is insignificant for an adult; naturally all quantities are cut in half for children. With two cups of Lobelia tea, a fever of 105 degrees that had raged for three days was broken in one half-hour!

And who is allowing the use of poisons? Consider that chlorine is a known factor in causing cancer in combination with other chemicals. Who permits it to be put in urban water supplies? Consider the use of lead in tin cans, often decried by the FDA but never completely prohibited! Consider the sale of liquor and tobacco products, heavily taxed for government profit but not prohibited! Consider the lavish use of sugar and salt, the two greatest chemical toxins allowed in our foods! Consider the permission to use powerful chemical preservative toxins, known to kill in larger amounts. Who is poisoning whom? Black pepper is another poison!

Headaches: can be relieved by taking a hot foot bath in water to which 2 tsp. of powdered mustard has been added. While soaking the feet for 10 to 20 minutes, apply a folded handkerchief to the head, well-dampened with equal parts of cold water and vinegar, renewing it frequently. Another old remedy is applying oil of rosemary to the temples and rubbing it in (caution: keep away from eyes!). Or another is to soak coarse brown paper in vinegar and plaster it on the forehead. As a mere pain remedy, white willow bark tea is safer than aspirin.

It should not be overlooked that most headaches come from tension, stress, overheating, blood pressure, or constipation. Removing those causes will usually banish the headache.

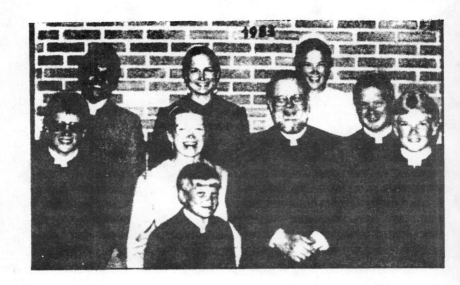

Chapter 3: *Recipes for the Reproductive System*

Shown above is a family picture of the author, his wife, and their seven unmarried children. Amish families regard children as assets, rather than liabilities. They may have as many as five to ten children. Their society does not dictate that they have to provide each with an expensive college education. Instead they are required only to equip each boy with a trade and each girl with the skills of being a homemaker.

For an Amish couple to be *childless* is regarded as a great tragedy. Theirs is still the Biblical view: "Thy wife shall be as a fruitful vine by the sides of thine house: thy children like olive plants round about thy table." (Psalm 128:3). "Lo, children are an heritage of the Lord: and the fruit of the womb is His reward. As arrows are in the hand of a mighty man, so are the children of the youth. Happy is the man that hath his quiver full of them!" (Psalm 127:3-5). For these reasons, the Amish are keenly interested in *family life* and concerned to reproduce themselves.

In May, 1984, the Amish family newspaper, *"The Sugarcreek, Ohio Budget"* contained an editorial report by the Associate Editor, George R. Smith, on a world record:

Amish Family Group Sets World Record

Large families have always been the rule among the Amish people and during my many years of association with The Budget I have made a list of some of the exceptionally large family groups mentioned in the obituary columns.

I had recorded two family groups of more than 500 members and thought my list was fairly complete until two weeks ago when Mrs. John D Schmucker Sr of Medford Wisc. reported the death of Adam Borntrager of that community and stated that he had 707 direct descendants, 675 of them still living.

This was such an astonishingly large total that I wrote to Mrs Schmucker, asking if that might include any adoptions, stepchildren, or any who were not blood relatives.

Here is her reply: Adam Borntrager, who died at age 96, had 11 children. 115 grandchildren, 529 greatgrandchildren, and 20 greatgreat-grandchildren, all living and all blood relatives. No adoptions or stepchildren In addition, 8 grandchildren and 24 great-grandchildren of the same family are deceased.

I felt that must be a world record so I consulted the Guiness Book of World Records and, sure enough. the largest family group recorded there was that of Mrs. Johanna Booysen of South Africa who was estimated to have 600 living descendants in January 1966, and Wilson Kettle of Newfoundland left 582 living descendants when he died in 1963 at the age of 102.

Up to this time, the largest Amish family group I had recorded was that of Bishop Moses Borkholder of Nappanee, Ind., who died in 1933 at the age of 94. He had 17 children by two wives. Eleven of the children survived him, along with 138 grandchildren, 388 great-grandchildren and 18 great-great-grandchildren; a total of 555 living descendants at the time he died.

Next the family of Jonas J. Schmucker of Geauga County. Ohio. Jonas died January 3, 1978 at the age of 90 years. At the time of his death he had 536 living descendants. He and his wife, the former Mary Ann D. Miller, had sixteen children. Fourteen of these children survived him, along with 130 grandchildren, 372 great-grandchildren and 20

great-great-grandchildren. However. 6 or 7 of the greatgrandchildren are adopted and cannot be considered direct descendants

Jonas was a native of Indiana. moving to Geauga County with his parents, Mr and Mrs. John S Schmucker at the age of thirteen His wife-to-be came to Geauga County with her parents, Dannie J Millers, from Holmes County just before the big snowstorm in April 1901

Then comes the family of John Eli Miller of Middlefield. who died in 1961 on the eve of his 95th birthday, leaving five of his seven children, 61 grandchildren, 338 great grandchildren and 6 great great grandchildren – a total of 410 living descendants at the time of his death. This is all the more remarkable when you consider that there were only seven children, and two of these died while comparatively young. During the last year of his life a new descendant was being born on an average of every ten days

Mr Miller married Sarah Schlabach in 1888 and she died in 1947 after 59 years of married life They moved from Holmes County to a new

community the Amish were then establishing near Middlefield in Geauga County. Ohio. Their first child was born in 1890 and seventy years later their descendants numbered over 400.

Mrs. Lydia Byler of Staunton, Va. celebrated her 96th birthday anniversary on April 14, 1983. At that time she had 486 living descendants. Eight of her ten children were still living, along with 60 grandchildren, 295 greatgrandchildren and 134 greatgreat-grandchildren. Perhaps someone can furnish more upto-date information on this family group.

To the best of my knowledge no other monogamous society in the world has recorded family groups as large as the Amish families mentioned above.

There probably are other Amish or Mennonite groups that I have overlooked. If so, I would be pleased if one of the descendants would supply me with as complete information as possible. This applies to the descendants of any man or woman now living, as well as any who are deceased.

George R. Smith
Associate Editor

All of this has a bearing on health. The statistics prove that married people live longer than those who are single, divorced or widowed. For example, married men live on an average of 5 years longer than bachelors. A man who kisses his wife in the morning before he leaves for work, is reported by the insurance companies to live an average of 5 years longer than those who do not! Affectionate ties with home guarantee a safer and longer life at home!

The *coronary thrombosis* death rate in Britain is 40% higher among widowers than among married men of the same age. Divorces are virtually unknown among the

Amish. Divorces are usually preceeded by tension, fighting, hostility, resentment, hardening of the heart, and *an unforgiving spirit,* all of which also cut down one's life! Long live the family!

Of course, the Amish concern for families is not just with *quantity* but with *quality.* To illustrate what differences different ideals can make over several generations, compare two family groups studied by sociologists: the Jukes and the Edwards.

Max Jukes lived in the state of New York. He did not believe in Christian training and married a girl of like character. From this union have come 1,026 descendants. 300 of then died prematurely; 100 were sent to the penitentiary for an average of 13 years each, and 100 became public prostitutes. There were more than 100 drunkards, and the whole family cost the state more than $1,200,000. They made little contribution to society.

Jonathan Edwards lived in the same state. He believed in Christian training and married a girl who had similar beliefs. From that union came 729 descendants. Out of this family have come 300 preachers, 65 college professors, 13 university presidents, 60 authors of good books, 3 U.S. Congressmen and one vice president of the U.S. The only black spot in the family was Aaron Burr, who married a girl of questionable character.

My own wife is a descendant of Jacob Hertzler, the first Amish bishop who came to America in 1749. By 1952, when a family history was written, there were 8,757 families of his descendants, including 36,548 individuals. Of these, 456 were ministers and bishops. There were 47 foreign missionaries, 74 nurses, 60 doctors and dentists, 64 college teachers and 7 college presidents, plus 523 other occupations.

It is a challenge to ask ourselves, what are we living for? If we are living for God and mankind, does He not promise blessings unto children's children? (Psalm 103:17-18).

Sterility: Two Amish home remedies for this are carrot seed oil and wheat germ oil. Both are vitamin rich. Daily consumption of carrot seed oil capsules has restored fertility. Wheat germ oil is another favorite. Eating a diet rich in alfalfa sprouts is also helpful. Abstaining from all working with insecticide sprays helped others to overcome sterility. Men should avoid wearing tight pants and underwear as tight clothing causes heat that cuts down the sperm count. Pumpkin seeds or a good zinc supplement is very helpful.

Impotence: After forty, men sometimes need an herbal supplement to their diet for tired glands. Most health food stores have an herb combination much used by the Amish containing Damiana, Siberian Ginseng, Echinacea, Fo-Ti, Gotu-Kola, Sarsaparilla and Saw Palmetto. Excellent teas effective for impotency are found in the author's new book on Indian Herbs.

Change of Life Stress: There is a hormone imbalance or cessation in the mid-life crisis for both men and women. The following herbs are used by the Amish with some success: Black·Cohosh, Sarsaparilla, Ginseng, Licorice, False Unicorn, Holy Thistle, Squaw Vine.

Pregnancy: Amish women tend to accept pregnancy as normal instead of as a "disease" or sickness. A common minor complication is **kidney trouble,** which they remedy with mild **diuretic teas** such as sweet fennel, watermelon seeds, parsley or bearberry to flush the kidneys.

Most Amish women take a special mixture 50-50 of Red Raspberry and Squaw Vine capsules 1-3 times a day through out the 9 month pregnancy or some prefer the loose tea leaves as it's cheaper. Then they use a last 6 weeks formula containing: Squaw Vine, Blessed Thistle, Black Cohosh, Penny Royal, False Unicorn, Red Raspberry Leaves, and Lobelia. Normal dosage is 1 capsule 3 times a day for the first month; second month, 2 capsules 3 times a day. Others take 2 capsules-3 times a day all six weeks. This is praised highly for faster and easier delivery. It prepares the birth canal giving elasticity to the pelvic and vaginal areas for easier delivery. The uterus is strengthened and less hemorrhaging! If they still have trouble, many have taken 2 capsules with a large glass of water, four times a day for 4 weeks, last 2 weeks they take 3 capsules 4 times a day. The above information is from testimonials from the Amish, but by no means is this a set standard for everyone.

Most morning sickness can be relieved by drinking red raspberry tea or a Pregancy Tea containing Spearmint Leaf, Strawberry Leaf, Alfalfa Leaf, Lemon Verbena, Lemon Balm, Nettle Leaf, Fennel Seed, Lemon Grass Leaf, Stevia Leaf and Red Raspberry Leaf.

Another good formula taken for both mother's and baby's sake is: Horsetail Grass, Oat Straw, Comfrey, Lobelia. This is a Natural Mineral Formula rich in silica, calcium, vitamin B-12 and trace minerals. It is helpful in problems such as: **broken and weak bones, falling hair, nail breaking, cramps in legs or muscles, calming nerves,** aiding **sleep,** building good **teeth** and preventing **cavities!**

Marshmallow or **Alfalfa Tea** is given to the mother to aid her milk supply. Another **Mother's Milk** Formula contains: Fennel Seeds, Spearmint Leaf, Coriander Seeds, Lemon Verbena, Anise Seed, Chamomile Flower, Borage Tops, Blessed Thistle Leaf, Althea Root, Lemon Grass Leaf, Stevia Leaf and Fenugreek Seed. It's good hot or iced!

Mothers with extra stress calm down with this EX-Stress formula: Black Cohosh, Cayenne, Hops Flowers, Mistletoe, Lobelia, Scullcap, Wood Betony, Valerian Root and Lady's Slipper.

A marvelous old Indian remedy used by Amish mothers who wish to prevent **miscarriage** and avoid painful and protracted labor, is to drink red raspberry leaf tea three times a day throughout the pregnancy (one half handful of the leaves to a cup of hot water). Others have gotten excellent results by taking a False Unicorn Combination containing: False Unicorn, Golden Seal Root, Squaw Vine and Orange Peel. The capsules usually gave good results! Others get quicker results by emptying 3 capsules in a cup which are steeped in boiling water.

Active farm mothers who keep on working at home generally have an easier delivery than those who give up all activity and grow fat and flabby.

Amish mothers tend to favor home births. Some have taken the Lamaze classes. Many have midwives attend them at home instead of bothering to go to hospitals for the increasingly expensive lying in care. If there are no complications in the birth, lengthy hospital stays are risky because of exposure to more germs. Some doctors advise caesarean section for convenience (and profit) rather than for any medical necessity. For these and other reasons, Amish mothers use hospitals less for births than the general public.

Post-partum hemorrhages are often stopped by administering an old herbal remedy called ergot. When my wife and I were teaching in Alaska years ago, I had to give an injection of ergotine to stop a severe case of bleeding. Teachers are authorized to act as medical assistants under doctor's direction but laymen should not give this drug. Shepherd's Purse given in capsule form or in extract form is also helpful in excessive bleeding.

Problems after birth: because of heavy mineral exhaustion and psychological stress, some mothers suffer post-partum depression. Spiritual counselling plus rebuilding with vitamin and mineral supplements is usually sufficient.

One mother with the problem of becoming almost **bald** with each pregnancy, was wonderfully helped by taking red clover tops tincture. Her hair came in thicker and more abundant than ever. 20 drops daily are used, for at least a month, drunk with a little water.

Breast problems: scanty flow of milk for nursing mothers is usually easily remedied by eating oatmeal gruel three times daily. Marshmallow herb and Blessed Thistle are also used here, plus drinking plenty of liquids. Alfalfa tea is used, too.

An ointment to dissolve **breast lumps** is made from equal parts of wintergreen oil, olive oil, and turpentine. Another Amish formula for the same problem is a liniment made from equal parts of pure castor oil and oil of wintergreen. Use only the *pure* wintergreen oil, not the synthetic imitation. The genuine thing can be purchased from Chupp's Herbs & Vitamins, 27539 Londick, Burr Oak, MI 49030-9746, as well as other hard to find herbs and vitamins. This also serves for lumps under the arm. Massage the lumps starting in the back and with fingers straight bring them across the affected area to the front. It is helpful to know that many breast lumps are caused by eating chocolate. 5 drops Brazilian Aveloz in cup Pau d' Arco tea 3 times a day has seen improvements on lumps, cysts, and tumors according to the new Indian Herb Book. It states not to use while pregnant. Users says it doesn't work for everyone.

Female troubles: under this euphemism, many problems were solved in times past by taking the popular Lydia Pinkham's Remedy. It was a compound of Licorice, Camomile, Pluerisy root, Jamaica dogwood, Black cohosh, Life plant and Dandelion root, in an alcohol tincture. It is used for the relief of symptoms of painful menstruation and change of life. If you cannot find it in your drugstore, your health food store will have alternative herbal combinations containing Golden Seal root, Blessed Thistle, Cayenne, Uva-ursi, Cramp bark, False Unicorn root, Raspberry leaves, Squaw vine, and Ginger.

Delayed menstruation: when there has been a cessation of the normal monthly flow, hot Ginger tea brings on menstruation. Another remedy for this is taking two cups of hot Camomile tea at one sitting. Another kind of tea much used for all kinds of menstrual complaints is Shave grass or Horsetail grass (rich in silica, a kidney cleanser).

Leukorrhea ("the whites"): this whitish discharge from the vagina can often be cleared up simply by administering a douche made of two teaspoonfuls of alum per quart of lukewarm water, or by two tablespoonfuls of ordinary white vinegar per quart of lukewarm water, used twice daily for one week.

Another old Amish recipe for **menstrual pains,** is to drink melissa tea with rue (½ tsp. of each herb, steeped for 10 minutes, strained).

An herb to **avoid** when *pregnant* or when wishing to become pregnant, is **pennyroyal.** I knew one young couple that had no children until they stopped drinking their daily ration of pennyroyal tea! **It discouraged conception.**

When the pregnancy term is *overdue*, there are two teas which are used to bring on labor almost immediately. But it should be emphasized that this works only when the baby is ready to come and this makes it easier and quicker! One cup of blue cohosh tea is drunk and then one cup of squaw vine tea.

During the last six weeks of pregnancy, many Amish women regularly take an herbal formula available in almost any health food store, which combines the following herbs in handy capsule form: Squaw vine, Blessed Thistle, Black Cohosh, Pennyroyal, False Unicorn, Red Raspberry Leaves, and Lobelia. You should not try to mix your own in this "six weeks' formula," because only a tiny amount of pennyroyal is usable. It is a great blessing that many traditional herbal combinations are available ready mixed and encapsulated in your health food stores. I suppose nowadays, Amish women using herbs are much more likely to use herbal combinations already in capsule form than to bother weighing out dried herbs and brewing teas. However, teas made from using herbs powdered in capsule form are also popular. The gelatin capsule is discarded and the herbal contents of three capsules are steeped in boiling water.

After the baby has come, and suffers from any *colic or stomach ache,* a favorite remedy is to give the baby either camomile tea or catnip tea. This acts as a calmative for baby (and mother, too!). Also a combination catnip and fennel has done wonders for babies with colic, minor pain, nerves, indigestion, stomach acid and gas. A few drops in tea or warm water taken orally or can be taken as an enema.

Prostate problems: Men, too, suffer various complaints peculiar to their sex. After forty, there are often congestions of the prostate gland. Prolonged congestion can lead to infection or even enlargement. This causes such symptoms as these: lower back pain, a heavy feeling of draggy tiredness, tenderness or swelling in the scrotum, interference with virility, and frequent urination yet leaving you with the feeling that you cannot empty your bladder.

Generations of Amish men have used the following simple remedies for this problem. Cut the corn silk from the tip of the sheath surrounding the corn cob, from a half dozen ears of corn; cook it into a tea and drink it three times daily for a week. Use fresh corn silk daily. We know of one Amish man who made himself a refreshing summer drink of corn silk tea and served it to his whole family daily like lemonade! It is a marvelous diuretic (cleanser of the whole genito-urinary tract). It is important to drink 2 glasses of water first thing in the morning to flush out toxins.

Pumpkin seeds are another remedy for this. The pumpkin seeds stimulate male hormone production and also act as a vermifuge or worm-killer. Peasants of all countries where pumpkins grow are familiar with this simple remedy to blitz internal parasites. A common veterinary medication for cows and chickens is extract of piperizina citrate, a pumpkin seed derivative. Some health food stores carry pumpkin seed oil, which may be taken in small amounts; chewing the fresh seeds is better. Also Pau d' Arco Tea several cups a day gave relief for most Amish men. Sometimes extra zinc is helpful, (this is taken from testimonials.) .

Seeds: These are nature's concentrated surprise packages, stuffed full of germinal life, overflowing with vitamins and minerals and containing many medicinal properties. Seeds too small to be chewed can be brewed into tea. [Be sure you use only untreated seeds, and that they are fresh or dried, but never rancid.] Here are some uses of seeds.

Watermelon seeds are a good kidney cleanser and prostate purge. Anise seed is a powerful diuretic, too; some chew it as a breath freshener after a meal. Fennel seed is useful in menstrual problems. Caraway seed is good for upset stomach. Burdock seed tea is a blood cleanser to banish boils and styes. Carrot seed oil capsules are good for improving *eyesight* and virility.

Sesame seeds have a laxative effect and also help prevent cholesterol congestion in blood vessels. Sesame seed candy was made in our home by taking the fresh sesame seeds and rolling them into a ball with honey, then freezing them to be eaten at leisure. Safflower seed oil is also used to lessen cholesterol congestion or plaque in blood vessels. Cardamom seeds are chewed to sweeten the breath. Flaxseed contains a healing oil called linseed oil (flax was used to make linen, so we have the name "lin(en)seed"). An ounce or two is first washed in cold water, then boiled and strained to make a cup of tea for a laxative. Hot flaxseed poultices are made by boiling in water, put mash on a clean, folded cloth, over sprains or chest congestions.

This chapter is on the *tree of life.* Every tree grows from a *seed.* The human reproductive system also produces "seed" from which a veritable tree of life or family tree grows, with branches to many generations. Be careful how you sow the seed. It was never meant to be wasted. In the spiritual sense, Amish believe that people need to be born again or born from above through the "seed" of Christ by the Word of God.

A beautiful Biblical symbol is the 7-branched lampstand called the *menorah* in the Old Testament. This was a stylized pattern of a tree or a plant. The 7-branched herb called *sage* (Salvia) or *moriah* in Hebrew may have been one of the original patterns. A picture of that plant is reproduced here. Also, the olive tree, whose leaves are green on top and silvery underneath, when a wind blows on them seems to shine and shimmer like light. Thus the "tree of life" was like a "lamp"!

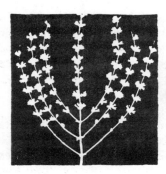

Zechariah 4:6 states that this tree-lamp is the Spirit and Word of God. Read Revelation 1:12-20.

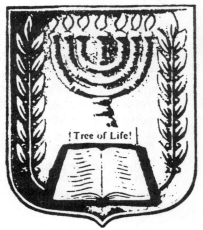

"Thy word is a lamp unto my feet, and a light unto my path." Psalm 119:105

! Tree of Life !

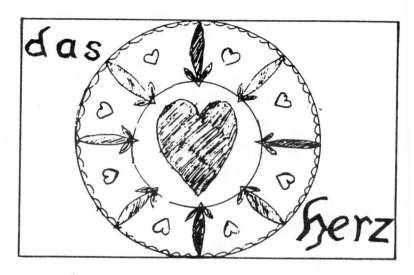

Chapter 4: **Recipes for Circulatory and Skeleto-Muscular System**

That heroic muscle of the body, the heart, tirelessly pumps the blood to nourish the whole system. Amish are as concerned as anybody in the general population with death from *heart and artery disease.* Too often, such death is unnecessary, a result of bad nutritional habits. The Amish, like Americans in general, are gradually becoming aware of the dangers of cholesterol, etc. Here they practice two simple remedies: apples reduce *cholesterol,* so many apples are eaten and much apple cider is drunk.

Recent European discoveries have proven that liberal use of garlic and onions will also reduce cholesterol plaque, triglycerides and related blood fats. The ancient Roman herbalist, Pliny (A.D. 23-79) recommended garlic for some 60 ailments, from the common cold to toothaches! Health-minded Amish eat an apple a day to keep the doctor away, and a garlic a day to keep everybody else away! The only real *danger with onions* is consuming two pounds daily will cause *low blood pressure, and thins the blood.* So be moderate!

Amish nutritionists like to point out that their favorite book, the Bible, long ago gave us clues as to what diet is good for the heart. Psalm 104:15 says: "bread...strengtheneth man's heart." According to Psalms 81:16 and 147:14, it is the "cream of the wheat" or "the fat of the wheat" which is its choicest ingredient. This has to refer to the vitamin E content of wheat germ. Unfortunately, modern milling techniques remove most of this vital nutrient and replace it with artificial additives to preserve "shelf-life" and increase profits.

Vitamin E has been discovered to be a powerful detoxifier, purging the arteries, decreasing blood clots, purifying the blood, increasing oxygen supply in the blood, and a help in avoiding the pains of angina pectoris which result from heart and blood starvation. Many Amish take from 100 to 300 units of vitamin E daily, or more. Safer yet is eating natural foods which are high in vitamin E. Here is a good Amish-Mennonite recipe for whole wheat bread:

Mildred Martin's Recipe for Whole Wheat Bread: Take 2 tblsp. dry yeast, 2 tsp. salt, ¼ cup honey, ¼ cup vegetable oil, one egg, and 4 cups of warm water; mix and let stand until yeast works. Add 12 to 14 cups of *only* fresh ground whole wheat flour, plus wheat germ for extra vitamin E and a nutty flavor; knead, let it rise; bake at 350 degrees. This makes three loaves.

A heart strengthening health diet will also avoid other cholesterol foods in excess: eggs, bacon, ham, butter, cheese, ice cream, milk (except for children), and chocolate. The Amish also protect their circulation by avoiding tight fitting fashionable clothes, belts and corsets, and instead wear comfortable, modest clothing with suspenders for men, and cool, long "granny" dresses for women.

Studies during the Viet Nam war showed that up to 65% of the American soldiers killed were already suffering from hardening of the coronary arteries. This is dietary suicide! But Vitamin C in large doses helps prevent arteriosclerosis. Safflower oil is also used by the Amish as a blood cleanser, to cut down cholesterol sludge. A good *heart tonic* is tea made from Hawthorn berries and cayenne (red pepper). Hawthorn berry extract leads to increased circulation in the coronary arteries, and tones the cardiac muscle.

Blood thinners: sassafras tea is a blood thinner (excessive amounts can lead to nose bleeds). Burdock, red clover tops and sassafras combined in a tea make a good blood cleanser.

An excellent blood cleanser which aids your *liver* and *gall bladder* contains Barberry Rt. Bark, Wild Yam, Cramp Bark, Fennel Seed, Ginger Rt., Catnip and Peppermint. 2 capsules taken before meals.

Exercise, in moderation, will not bring on a heart attack, rather it helps you to avoid one. Walk at least one mile daily. Blood clots form rather when blood flow is sluggish. More than 50% of heart attacks take place while the victim is sleeping! So walk and climb unless you want to die on "coronary hill" from a 'rusty' heart! A mini trampoline in the home can give the needed exercise.

Blood circulation: can be improved by drinking a combination tea of Rosemary and camomile, one cup hot before retiring. This will help poor circulation in the lower limbs and cold feet. Some Amish put powdered red pepper (cayenne) in their stockings and gloves to warm cold extremities in winter. This improves circulation, too.

Phlebitis: Take 1 tsp. safflower oil before breakfast; 3 garlic oil capsules daily before meals, and 3 cups of alfalfa seed tea daily (crush 2 tsp. of seeds, soak them in boiling water). A good salve to put on phlebitis: elevate the affected limb and gently apply at or on the hurt place a salve made from Ginseng, Aloe Vera, Allantoin, A, D, E, and B-6. This salve can be bought ready made in most health food stores. I remember how it worked for a young Amish man who had spent days in the hospital but had not been helped until he used this salve, then he was soon cured.

Bone decay salve: Here is a case history using a traditional Amish salve for "white swelling" or bruised and infected bones. A 23 year old soldier was involved in an accident in which a heavy weight dropped on the front of his lower right leg, breaking the skin and badly bruising the bone. Infection set in and the doctors decided to amputate after massive antibiotics failed to help. The young man pled with them to *wait*. He wrote to his parents in Ohio to contact an Amish herbalist for help.

I spoke later to the Amish herbalist, Sim Schlabach, who had this recipe from his ancestor, Hans Plank, the Amish herb doctor who came to America in 1752. Take 1 lb. finely pulverized rosin, 1 lb. mutton tallow shaved fine, 2 oz. sweet oil (pure olive oil), 2 oz. granulated sugar pulverized; mix all ingredients *cold* (do not heat); apply three times daily. The young soldier got the salve and had a friendly nurse apply it to his leg. Whenever the doctors were going to inspect the leg, the nurse carefully wiped away the salve so they would not know what was being done. In two weeks the leg was perfectly healed! The doctors congratulated themselves on this case of spontaneous remission! [What the doctor doesn't know doesn't hurt him!] Later the young soldier and the nurse were married!

Backache: Don't eat eggs, beef, pork or cheese and many a stubborn case of chronic back ache will clear up. Fat-heavy diet is the cause of much kidney and back pain. Also a good calcium supplement has helped many. One also can take Willard Water and put in distilled water and use that as drinking water.

Drawing salve: Take a lump of each of these ingredients, the size of an egg: hog's lard, beeswax, rosin, and hard brown laundry soap shaved fine; heat all slowly in an iron kettle, dissolve, pour into a jar and cool until hard. This will clean up **carbuncles,** draw **poison** matter. Amish call it Zeeg-schmeer. Another good formula available at Health Food Stores is: Chaparral, Comfrey, Red Clover Blossoms, Pine Tar, Mullein, Beeswax, Plantain, Olive Oil, Mutton Tallow, Chickweed, Poke Root. It's also used on ulcers, tumors, boils, warts, skin cancers and hemorrhoids. Excellent for burns and as a healing and drying agent.

Brant schmeer: Here is another healing salve recipe from Sim Schlabach. It is used for **skin cancers** and **blood poisoning.** Take hog's lard without salt, ½ gal. Put the lard in a large kettle and heat it; then drop in a large handful of fresh green rue and let it grow brown; then add 7 to 9 eggs beaten up. When it gets dark brown, discard the herbs and cool. I got this recipe from Sim Schlabach when he was 90 years old, still hale and hearty. He was a great-great-great-grandson of Hans Plank (whose daughter married Strong Jacob Yoder and passed the cures down to her descendants).

Cancer formula: Here is another priceless formula that may save lives. It is translated from a German writing owned by Eli M. Kuhns (by Leroy Beachy in 1981). A "sure remedy for cancer removal without surgery, causes very little pain." Take 1 lb. figs and boil them slowly in 1 gal. fresh cow's milk until they are soft. Then remove them from the milk and place them in a jar, stirring them with a long fork until it has the consistency of a salve. Apply a plaster of this salve and drink of the milk every 12 hours for as long as you wish. The cancer should break open in 24 to 48 hours. If it does not, it is too far advanced (if internal, such as in stomach or female organs, nothing can be done). This formula goes ultimately back to one used in Bible times by Isaiah; read Isaiah 38:21 and II Kings 20:7.

Blood-poisoning: An antiseptic powder is made from one

part sulphur, one part alum and one part gun-powder. Sim Schlabach said you should put as much as will lay on a dime into water with a little vinegar, and give it once an hour for 3 hours internally, then after that three times daily as long as necessary for blood poisoning. You may also sprinkle it externally on broken skin. (For gangrene it is used internally.) (Use it cautiously.)

Bruises: Crush a handful of fresh peach leaves and apply like a poultice to bruises.

Blood builder: One part of red beet juice to two parts of red grape juice; take 1 tblsp. three or four times daily. Beet Powder capsules are easier to take.

Antiseptic soak: For any open sore or cut, soak it in a solution of 2 or 3 tbsp. hardwood ashes to 1 gal. water, as hot as can be endured. Soak day and night. One may also apply Willard Water.

Blood poison: Take a pan of hot ashes; it could even contain some live coals. Sprinkle it heavily with sugar, dampen it, place the affected limb over the fuming pan, and cover everything with a woolen cloth. Take care not to burn the part but fumigate well.

Pain liniment: Dissolve 24 aspirins in 1 quart of rubbing alcohol. Rub on liberally for any ache; also good for tired feet. White or Red Tiger Balm from China is very effective. Red is the strongest.

Boils: Among children, on arms, legs, chest, etc., make a whipped potpourri of 4 oz. sublimed sulphur mixed with 16 oz. honey; take internally 1 tsp. at bedtime. Black Ointment applied on boils is helpful. A good blood cleanser like Red Clover Blossom extract should be taken also.

Boils in adults: Take 3 drops turpentine on 1 tsp. sugar once a day for three days, then wait three days and repeat; also put a couple drops externally (without rubbing) of equal parts of oil of turpentine, olive oil, oil of wintergreen and vinegar. In a few days it should dry up Another good recipe is to take equal parts of raw linseed oil and honey and enough flour to make a paste, and apply it to the boil or carbuncle. (Don't use boiled linseed oil from the hardware, but *raw*.) Here is another old remedy: keep a piece of pork rind and fat in a jar in your medicine cabinet; it can be kept for years even though rancid; apply it to a boil to draw it out. Also the latter two formulas for children help adults also. Chaparral capsules are helpful.

Bruises, aches, pains: Here is the formula for what is called "Good Samaritan Oil". Blend into 1 quart of raw linseed oil the following: ¼ oz. oregano oil, ¼ oz. oil of hemlock, ½ oz. oil of sassafras, ¼ oz. oil of wintergreen, ¼ oz. oil of lavender, 1 oz. gum camphor. Gently rub it in.

Finger-pressure massage: Known for centuries in Japan as Shiatsu; many Amish practice massage by applying simple thumb and hand pressure on various zones of the body. (Some use an acupuncture chart. Scientists have recently discovered that there is electrical activity along the traditional acupuncture lines, so this is not something occult or superstitious.) Amish practitioners of massage often speak of having the experience of massaging painful parts, then "feeling the pain" transferred to their own hands, so that they shake them afterwards or wash them vigorously. Many practice giving "foot-treatments," massaging various areas of the feet to relieve pain elsewhere in the body. This is sometimes called "reflexology." In any case, skilled massage is a great pain reliever, especially around the head and neck to relieve tension headaches.

Headaches: A liniment is made from sweet spirit of nitre (92% alcohol, ethyl nitrite 17½ gr. to the oz.) and rubbed externally. 1 tsp. of each: spirits of nitre, spirits of turpentine, and oil of juniper, blended together, make an Amish home remedy for **lumbago**; they take 9 drops of this mixture on a level tsp. of sugar once a day before retiring. It causes sweating and sometimes heart palpitations. A well known herb, White Willow Bark, has helped many.

Blood poisoning: Here is another remedy. Peach leaves, brewed into a strong brew (using 20 leaves per quart pan), is used to *bathe* an infected arm or leg; apply hot. Within 10 minutes of the application, sometimes the streaks come back down the arm! [*Note: Do NOT drink.*]

Arthritis: Often this is due to food poisoning from overeating foods in the deadly nightshade family (potatoes, tomatoes, green peppers, egg plant). There is a green dye in unripe or spoiled portions of these plants that 5 parts in a million is enough to make you stiff. While we lived in Costa Rica, I ate many potatoes which had green sunscald spots on them. I soon got to the place where I could not even walk and had to be in a wheel chair. Medical doctors simply declared, after two weeks in the hospital, that I had "rheumatoid arthritis" and would be a life-long invalid! The only thing I could do would be to take up to 25 aspirins per day for the pain!

Unwilling to accept such idiotic advice, I prayed for better guidance and was led to herbs and diet as a means of detoxifying my body. I drank lots of carrot juice, which really flushed out many poisons from my system. I took homeopathic herbs for arthritis (Bryonia, Rhododendron and Poison Ivy—these are so diluted that they cannot hurt but full strength these herbs would kill you). In two months I was normal again, thank God! A good Yucca combination in capsule form contains Yucca, Comfrey Root, Chaparral, Alfalfa, Burdock Root, Buckthorn Bark, Black Cohosh Root, Parsley, Slippery Elm Bark, Yarrow, Chelated Trace Minerals, Cayenne and Lobelia. For quicker results some Amish take Devil's Claw Caps with other remedies.

Sciatic rheumatism: Take 100% pure juice of aloe vera and drink 3 ounces, three times a day, while fasting. If the juice gripes your stomach, buffer it with a little olive oil each time you take it. Pains should soon diminish and then disappear. Many Amish sell this juice. It comes from a healing desert succulent plant.

Chaparral: This is another healing desert shrub. It contains a natural plant chemical which stifles the growth of other plants near it. We use it in ointment form to put on skin cancers. As a tea, dried chaparral leaves have been used for cancer by southwestern Indians.

Tennis shoulder: Buy avocadoes in the grocery store and horse tail grass in the herb store; take 4 avocado seeds and chop them, add them with 3 oz. horse tail grass to a quart of water and cook down to 1 pint. Then add 1 pint of rubbing alcohol and bottle. Used as a liniment, it should instantly cure.

Avocado: This is a very healing tree. After we eat the fruit, we save the large seed and sprout it by suspending it in a jar of water, just under the surface. After it roots, we plant it in pots. They make nice ornamental house plants. The avocado leaves are a very good home remedy with which to make tea (3 leaves per cup); this tea is good for dissolving *kidney stones.* A good tea for diabetes is to take three cups daily of the tea made by boiling ¼ avocado leaf, 1 eucalyptus leaf and 1 walnut leaf. It has cured some of *diabetes.*

Sciatic rheumatism: another remedy. Magdalena Graber cured herself of this ailment by taking 6 oranges, 6 lemons, and 6 grapefruit, cutting them up, cooking them (peeling and all) in two quarts of water; strain and add ¼ cup epsom salts; let it cook down to one quart, and then stand overnight. Take 1 tblsp. 3 times daily.

Broken bones: heal faster if you drink comfrey tea 3 times daily plus bone meal tablets. A good bone, flesh and cartilage builder has a combination of herbs: White Oak Bark, Comfrey Root, Marshmallow Root, Mullein, Black Walnut Hulls, Gravel Root, Wormwood, Lobelia and Scullcap.

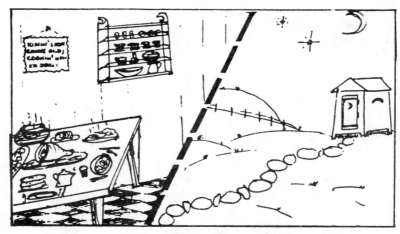

Chapter 5: **Recipes for the Digestive System**

Just as the last chapter could be subtitled "the Blood of life" because of its focus on circulation, so this chapter could be subtitled "the Bread of life." We are interested in real *LIFE* and health, *vitality* rather than merely existing. Yet as we study remedies for the digestive system, we must remember *"man cannot live by bread alone."* Sickness is often not only from what you eat, *but also from what is eating you!*

A healthy diet is a balanced diet. The first vital nutrient that is being mishandled in the average American diet is *water*. Much sickness from body toxins can be traced to constipation from inadequate water intake. Country people like the Amish are generally healthy because they **drink plenty of water.** You should have at least 6 glasses daily.

We drink water in teas, fruit and vegetable juices, soups and by the water-glass! Water aids circulation, metabolism, and elimination, as well as digestion. Sprinkle a pinch of vitamin C powder in glass of water to neutralize nitrates and toxins.

Roughage: Another missing ingredient for most people's digestion is sufficient roughage. An effete civilization likes soft breads, gooey desserts, and ground up main courses! You can, however, see the Amish walking around munching on raw celery and carrot sticks, eating their fruit unpeeled, their potatoes with the jackets on them, crunchy nuts, leafy vegetables, homemade cereals. All of these help supply the bulk needed to stimulate peristaltic movements in our alimentary canal!

Recipe for Crunchy Amish Cereal: Take 6 cups of oatmeal, 1 cup of coconut shredded, 3 cups of wheat germ, ½ cup of chopped almonds, ½ cup of chopped pecans, 1½ cups brown sugar, ½ tsp. salt, ½ cup vegetable oil; mix in big bowl and toast in the oven until crunchy.

Drying foods: Amish like to eat parched corn, dried apples; dried bananas, home-made raisins, dried peaches. All of these are favorite snacks. For centuries Amish families have had "schnitz" frolics to dry foods.

Laxative teas: Bulk without irritation is supplied by flaxseed and psyllium seed; 1 heaping tsp. of either seed, steeped in a cup of boiling water, cooled, is drunk for giving mucilaginous bulk. Senna leaf tea is a favorite laxative.

Abdominal pain: Chew well and swallow a tsp. of flaxseed. Or apply a rag wet with kerosene over the appendix, then cover it with a towel and a hot water bottle. See the doctor for acute abdominal pain.

Amoebas: These parasites abound in the tropics. When we lived there we learned of three good remedies (besides the precaution of always boiling or filtering your drinking water) a tea made of the bark of a mango tree, grind up a portion of the bark on the west side of the tree, boil 1 tsp. for tea. Or eat one papaya leaf per day to protect and cure yourself from amoebas. Or take 3 to 6 garlic caps daily. Garlic also equalizes **blood pressure.**

Canker sores: a symptom of hyperacidity. Avoid all soda pop. Make a mouth wash of 1 tsp. powdered myrrh, 1 tsp. golden seal, and 1 tsp. cayenne pepper; blend this into 1 quart water, rinse mouth frequently.

Constipation: Use more water and more roughage; try senna leaf tea or Pau d' Arco Tea. Magnesium is usually lacking, also exercise.

Colitis: Take comfrey and fenugreek capsules, or marshmallow, Slippery Elm, Comfrey Root, Lobelia, Ginger, Wild Yam combination.

Diabetes: See the tea mentioned on page 45 . Also good is a tea made from peach leaves. One man we know of took 3 cups of peach leaf tea daily (1 leaf per cup) and no longer needed to take his daily insulin shot. We know of several people who cured themselves of diabetes by making a tea of the cheese plant (marshmallow, in Dutch called kase-poppala) leaves. Some use it to control their diabetes without insulin. Another remedy is to take herbal combination capsules containing Cedar Berries, Uva Ursi, Licorice Root, Mullein, Cayenne and Golden Seal Root. The Amish use strawberry leaf tea to reduce sugar count. H. Zeis was using Pau d' Arco and it so happened that his sugar count went from 156 to 116.

Drunkenness: The infallible "cure" is prevention by total abstinence. Swallowing a small measure of olive oil before drinking is another remedy.

Diarrhea: An old remedy is slippery elm. We always use blackberry juice, too. Another recipe is to brew tea from dried blackberry roots. Red Raspberry Leaf tea or White Oak Bark is also helpful.

Dry mouth and throat for speakers: Great-grandpa Simon Hartzler, a Sunday-school teacher, chewed small pieces of dried calamus-root.

Flatulence (gas): Hot ginger tea, homemade ginger ale, or even ginger capsules are good for this condition. Or, you may chew a tsp. full of caraway seeds (or coriander seeds). Drink warm mint tea. Eat slowly, do not bolt your food. Avoid all carbonated drinks. Another good formula is: Fennel, Wild Yam, Catnip, Ginger, Peppermint, Spearmint, Papaya and Lobelia. Take capsules at meal time as needed.

Gall bladder trouble: Mrs. Evelyn Kropf uses the juice of 3 lemons, 3 tsp. of cream of tartar, and 3 tsp. of epsom salts, put in a pint jar of water; take 1 tbsp. of the solution in the morning before breakfast. Or try 1 tsp. of olive oil, followed by 1 tsp. of lemon juice, three times daily for three days, fasting.

Annie Mendel, a famous Hutterite bonesetter, uses lemon and olive oil for gall bladder. We have even seen kidney stones passed when ½ cup of olive oil was drunk with lemon.

Gout: For drawing soreness from gout affected toes or feet, chop raw onions and apply as a poultice, leaving on one day. Eating daily a couple cups of fresh cherries and a meatless diet helps. Yucca and Devil's Claw capsules help also.

Pinol (pine oil solution) was used to add to bath water to make a refreshing, relieving bath for gout sufferers. Also the affected limb was later wrapped in heated wool to induce perspiration.

Offensive breath: Chew pieces of sweet calamus root (pare off root bark first). Another remedy is to take purified charcoal tablets; they cleanse the stomach and intestines of foulness. Also a lower bowel cleanser taken for at least 3 months helped some.

Piles: Make a tea from sumac tops and drink before retiring and first thing in the morning. Also gently steam the affected parts by sitting over a pan containing garlic boiled in milk; let the vapors rise. Jimson weeds, fried in lard, make a good ointment to spread on piles. Some have found relief by going on a grape fast, with only grape juice taken for seven days.

Hyperacidity: Most Americans are too acid. This disorders the entire metabolism, and even affects the personality. Too many are of a sour and bitter disposition, "sour grapes have set their teeth on edge." Attention should be given to including more alkaline foods in the diet (apples and carrots, for example) and avoiding acid drinks (soda pop, coffee, liquor). Calcium and magnesium tablets are good antacids.

Hemorrhoids: Another old-timey remedy is soaking in a hot sitz-bath to which a pound of alum has been added. A good ointment containing Marigold, Malva, Comfrey, Red Clover, Burdock, Elder and Yellow Dock gives relief many times.

Stomach cancer: One of the great meadow plants brought by the Pennsylvania Dutch to improve the American soil was the red clover. Like alfalfa, it is a powerful concentration of vitamins and minerals. A tea made of red clover tops has been employed for centuries in combatting the ravages of cancer. Also available in the better health food stores is the liquid extract of red clover tops. We take 10 to 20 drops of this every morning.

Ulcers: Drink cabbage juice, 6 oz., a half hour before meals. If you don't have a juicer, put 3 cups of chopped cabbage and 16 oz. water in the blender on chop, then strain and drink. Cabbage contains vitamin U. Aloe Vera Juice also is healing.

Vomiting: To stop nausea, drink a tea made from peach leaves. **CAUTION!** Use only **one** leaf per cup! Red Raspberry tea is also helpful.

50

Worms: Garlic capsules discourage all but the most hearty worms. Health food stores also have an anti-parasite syrup that is very effective. It is compounded of fennel seed, black walnut hulls, senna leaves, male fern, tansey, tame sage, and wormwood. Another old Amish remedy is a tea made from pumpkin seeds (remove outer shell and toast the seeds).

Weight control: The general public thinks of the Amish as a very austere people. While it is true we strive for simplicity in many areas of life, to our shame we are tempted much to sin at the table. Someone has said, "Appetite is the last sin to be overcome."

The Amish are hearty workers, and hearty eaters. The best cure for gluttony is do "Push-ups," that is, to push yourself up from the table! *Temperance* or self-control in eating and drinking is just as much a part of religion as any other virtue. It is necessary at times to go on a partial fast. We especially like the *juice fast* system. I lost 30 pounds and eliminated great amounts of toxins by drinking carrot juice 4 and 5 times daily for two weeks. Don't be alarmed if your skin starts to turn orange, this is only a carotene tint and will go away.

An Amish lady in PA (letter on file) wrote that by taking 2 Chickweed capsules before meals and 2 capsules of this weight loss formula: Chickweed, Saffron, Burdock, Parsley, Kelp, Licorice, Fennel, Echinacea, Black Walnut, Papaya, Hawthorn Berries and Mandrake she lost 18 lbs. the first month and lost another 20 lbs. reaching her goal. She didn't eat any sweets or baked products, pastries etc., and cut down her eating., She had energy to spare and soreness and pain in her feet disappeared! One who eats only raw fruits and vegetables will lose weight faster. She also took a multi-vitamin daily. Many get good results drinking a Chinese Slim tea.

For *overweight,* a tea is prepared from the orange berries

of the mountain ash tree. The berries are dried and 1 tsp. used per cup, without sweetening of any kind.

The grape juice fast has been used by many. One lady suffering from ovarian cancer that had spread to her kidneys was able to overcome it by abstaining from all other food and drink, while she drank three 24 oz. bottles of grape juice daily for two weeks. During that time corruption just oozed from her body. Doctors pronounced her cured, unable to understand what had dissolved the cancer.

Underweight: Thin persons suffering lack of appetite and general lassitude are much strengthened by taking 10 drops of liquid red clover tops extract, three times daily. This plant is a chief regulator of the metabolism and besides a blood purifier and general detoxifier. As the Germans say: *Guten Appetit!* (Good appetite!).

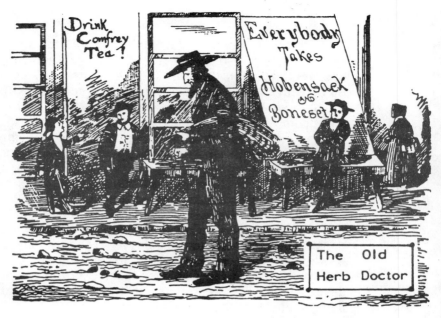

Drink Comfrey Tea!

Everybody Takes Hobensack or Boneset

The Old Herb Doctor

Chapter 6: *Recipes for the Respiratory System*

We could subtitle this chapter, "the Breath of life." As we breathe in the life-giving oxygen and breathe out the carbon dioxide wastes, we are taking our part in the world's air cycle. Trees and plants absorb the carbon dioxide and respire oxygen for us. We all participate in a gaseous exchange to sustain the environment.

It is sad that there is so much industrial air pollution and cigarette smoking. Polluted air is defined as 2,000 particles of pollution in a section of air half the size of a sugar cube. When the pollution level reaches 35,000 particles, it is fatal for humans. Some cities average 15,000 particles already! Sad!

Pneumotherapy or respiratory therapy is the study of methods of improving the quality of our respiration. The

Bible compares our physical respiration with the need of our spiritual man to live by the Holy Spirit: "that which is born of the Spirit is spirit" (John 3:6). Jesus compares the Holy Spirit with the wind blowing invisibly yet visibly affecting us. In olden times, when a man was hovering between life and death, a mirror would be placed to his lips to see if vapor condensed on it, showing he was still living. The Bible says, "What is your life? It is even a vapor, that appeareth for a little time, and then vanisheth away." (James 4:14). *Pneuma* means both breath and spirit.

It is now thought that insufficient vitamin C is likely to be the decisive contributing factor when arteries begin to degenerate. Dr. Emil Ginter discovered that a daily dose of less than 1000 mg. of vitamin C lowers the blood level of cholesterol by about 10%, when taken over the course of 47 days. Vitamin E protects against the air pollution toxins in smog that inhibit our respiratory enzymes.

So respiratory therapy begins with vitamin protection! It continues with learning better methods of breathing. Most people have shallow breathing instead of the healthier deep breathing. Amish are a fresh-air rural folk. They know it is important to live in well-ventilated houses, with the rooms aired out. Even the wash is dried in the sun and the wind and the air.

Musty, moldy houses are places that breed disease. Even attics and basements should be well-ventilated and dehumidified. In Bible times, incense of aromatic herbs was burned to fumigate buildings from decay and disease. The ancient Greeks and Romans used more than 150 different herbs for inhalation therapy (*per fume* means "by smoke"). Amish today also use vaporizers and inhalers to get the benefits of aromatic herbs.

For example, for *colds* and stuffy noses, we use a vaporizer at night with oil of peppermint or spearmint for decongestion. Pine oil, cedar oil and mint oil cut down air bacteria count. Europeans have long known that a sanitorium in an evergreen forest is more conducive to recuperation. Russian hospitals discovered that merely by placing potted pine trees in hospital rooms, they were able to reduce the bacteria count in the air. (Floors should be scrubbed with pinesol or pinol solutions.)

For *stuffy nose,* many Amish use the Olbas inhaler from Switzerland, containing oils of menthol, peppermint, cajeput and eucalyptol. This is safer than the American-made inhaler which has petroleum products or harsh chemicals. Breathing in peppermint oil fumes also helps.

Medical malpractise dangers: It remains a frightening fact but true that many modern drugs have dangerous side-effects. There is absolutely no scientific cure for the common cold. Reckless use of antibiotics has even made pneumonia once again an important source of deaths; super strains of pneumonia have mutated on a diet of haphazard antibiotics given to people with colds!

A medical doctor friend of mine recently wrote me: "Being raised Amish, I know of many remedies my mother used to use. When in Switzerland for a medical convention, I heard a noted pediatrician speak of the efficacy of the old-fashioned onion poultice for children whith chest colds, even *pneumonia,* rather than so-called antibiotics which can be unsafe in their side-effects. In fact, I had a man in the office this morning who was suffering from liver damage following a prolonged use of antibiotics."

Aureomycin has caused death, liver damage, and internal bleeding. Chloromycetin has been known to induce fatal shock, double vision and blood disease. Cortisone and ACTH have caused perforated ulcers, shock and death. Streptomycin has caused abcesses, deafness, delirium and madness. Suphonamides have even caused kidney damage, sterility, cardiac damage, insanity and death. Patient beware!

Asthma: One of the hardest allergies to overcome. Often a child will first have eczema or hayfever, then asthma. I had it as a child, outgrew it, and then got it again in later life when under considerable stress. It makes you feel so helpless! Thank God it is not incurable. I got over mine by diet and herbs. Here are some suggestions.

Breathe Easy tea found in Health Stores is good to take with any breathing problems.

A good asthma syrup contains Comfrey Root, Mullein, Garlic, Fennel Seed, and Lobelia in Vegetable Glycerine and Apple Cider Vinegar.

A good chest and lung tonic combination contains: Marshmallow, Mullein, Comfrey, Lobelia and Chickweed.

A seven year old Amish girl was cured of *asthma* by using Lugol's iodine solution (available from a drug store): 5 drops in a half glass of milk twice daily for two weeks, then skip 2 weeks and repeat until cured.

A 25 year old Amish man was cured of severe asthma by taking 4 tblsp. of aloe vera gel daily for 2 weeks; take this before meals and bedtime.

Acute asthma attack: Steep 4 oz. powdered lobelia in 1 quart of rum; let it stand for 7 days, then strain. Take ½ tsp. during an attack. Some use this daily as a preventive, using 3 drops 3 times daily.

Asthma program: Eliminate all highly refined foods such as sugar, flour and homogenized milk, coffee, black tea, soda pop and chocolate. Avoid all dusts and powders and pollens. Get the following herbal combination in capsule form: marshmallow, mullein, comfrey, lobelia, and chickweed. Take 3 caps 3 times daily.

Bronchitis: Use mustard plaster, applied to chest and back as often as necessary. This is made from powdered black

56

mustard, 1 tblsp. mustard to 4 tblsp. flour. Mix in bowl, make a runny paste, fold between two large handkerchiefs and apply. (Oil skin first with a little olive oil if patient is sensitive.) Keep changing these mustard plasters as congestion lessens.

Bronchial coughs: An Amish man had such coughs that he thought he would never get his breath, until he took a piece of ginseng root, chewed it up, and was cured. Elderberry tincture also is good for coughs.

Bad colds: Make this salve and apply to chest, or for earaches. Take 6 oz. sheep tallow, 15 oz. vaseline, 3 oz. menthol crystals, 3 oz. beeswax, melt and add 2 ox. gum camphor oil, 2 oz. sassafras oil, 2 oz. eucalyptus oil. Apply liberally. (—Mrs. Levi Miller). Vitamin C powder seems to take down infection.

Children should sit with their feet in a pan of hot tea made from Queen Anne's lace, while they have a wool blanket over their shoulders and body. They should also drink elder blossom tea.

Choking: If the obstruction cannot be dislodged by thumping on the back or turning upside down, break an egg into a cup and have the patient swallow it.

Croup: Drink a tea made with slippery elm bark and horehound. Or: take onions, peel and slice them, fry them until brown, and place between two large men's handkerchiefs and apply to the patient's chest, *an onion poultice!* Po Ho oil is helpful.

Cough drops: Take 1 oz. cubeb powder, 2 oz. gum arabic, 2 oz. licorice root powdered, 1 lb. powdered sugar and mix with 4 tblsp. of water. You might also add some powdered charcoal (1 tsp.). —Simon Hartzler.

Cough syrup: To a tumbler full of honey, add 7 drops of eucalyptus oil and stir well. Take a few drops each time.

Take 1 lb. of fresh garlic and cut it into slices. Pour 1 quart of boiling water over it and let it stand in a covered vessel for 12 hours. Add a little bruised caraway and fennel seed, boiled for a short time in vinegar (this will mask the garlic smell). Strain and add honey to make a syrup.

Croup: If you are not squeamish, and want to cure croup in children, take 15 live bees and squeeze them to death, then put them in a pot and pour ½ pint of boiling rain water over them. Cover and let stand for 8 minutes. Strain out the bees and squeeze liquid out of them once more, through a cloth, into the water, then discard them. Take 1 tsp. of this every ½ hour. Also rub the chest, back and throat with goose fat.

Earache: An old remedy is to dip cotton in molasses and put it in the ear for pain. Oil of Herbs: a few drops in ear. *Acute earache:* Try otagesine, available at Health Stores.

In general, you should not put anything smaller than your elbow into your ear! However, a drop of oil of rue plus several drops of warm olive oil will often help earache. Warm smoke blown into the ear will often calm pain. Smoke should be from burning either tobacco or lobelia.

Eyes: Growth of cataracts can be retarded by dropping 1 drop of raw linseed oil in eyes at bedtime.(—Martha Varner). Camomile tea, dropped warm (not hot) into the eyes will cure styes. If you have a tiny irritant in the eye, put a single flaxseed under the eyelid. It will swell up and draw the irritant to itself. Catalyst altered water-spray on eyes seems to help.

Flu: Elderberry flowers make a good tea for the flu. A good compostition tea for colds and flu is made with ¼ tsp. of cinnamon and ¼ tsp. of cayenne in a cup of hot water. It will really make you sweat! (—Roy Strubhar).

A good flu combination is Bayberry Bark, Ginger Root, Cloves, Cayenne and White Pine Bark.

Another good composition tea for *colds and flu* comes from Gabe Brunk: take 1 lb. bayberry bark, 1 lb. hemlock bark, 1 lb. ginger root, 2 oz. cayenne pepper, and 2 oz. cloves. All ingredients must be finely pulverized and well-mixed. Use ¼ tsp. of this composition and 1 tsp. of sugar, put in a cup and pour boiling water over it. Let it stand for a few minutes and drink warm.

Another good one for *earaches:* mix several drops of glycerin with 4 % carbolic acid, warm; put in the ear.

Another old-fashioned cough syrup is made just from mullein leaves. Wash and clean the leaves, boil and then strain. Add enough sugar and cook down to a thick syrup.

Gargle: Apple cider vinegar is an effective throat gargle(—David Peachey). Another is to take 1 tblsp. sage leaves, a chunk of alum big enough to be bitey, and 1 tsp. 20 Mule Team Borax, add them to one pint of water, boil, let it settle, and gargle!

Another one for gargle: gargle with sumac tea. Gargle with salt water as hot as you can bear it.

Goiter: An iodine liniment to relieve goiter is made from 12 drams of iodide of potassium flakes, 6 drams of iodine (flakes), 3 grams of camphor, and put into 12 oz. of rubbing alcohol, and 12 oz. of water of ammonia. Apply externally once a day, in the evening. A druggist could compound this for you. Takes time to work. A good herbal combination is: Kelp, Dulse, Iris Moss, and Parsley, Mullein, Watercress, Lobelia.

Hiccups: Put one third tsp. of cream of tartar in a glass of warm water, drink three or four times a day on an empty stomach. Also this is good for a weak stomach. —Elmer Miller. Pull on tip of tongue or eat 1 tsp. peanut butter.

Another common hiccup remedy is to hold your breath for a time. Or take the juice of half an orange.

Hoarse throat: An old Amish remedy for hoarse song leaders is to chew a piece of ginseng root. As it dissolves it will clear up your throat. Olba's Oil is good also.

Honey remedies: Here are two testimonies for the healing power of honey. Melvin S. Fisher reports that he had a bad burn on his hand from a torch. After a scab formed he applied honey twice daily and in a short time it healed without a scar. Mrs. Fausnight reports how a lady had stepped on a nail and it went through her shoe sole. Blood poisoning set in and the doctor wanted to amputate. An old friend advised to put a honey poultice on the wound, wrapping it up. By the next morning, the honey had drawn out a small piece of leather! The foot was saved. Honey will also help soften up splinter soreness, so the splinters can be removed.

Mucus: Fenugreek tea removes mucus. Mucus is provoked by an overacid diet as well as by allergies. Avoid flour, sugar, and acid drinks. A good herbal combination is Fenugreek and Comfrey.

Nasal catarrh: In olden times, people regularly snuffed a handful of salt water up their nostrils each morning to clear the nose. Inhaling aromatic vapor from steaming spearmint will quickly clear you nose and sinus.

Pink-eye: Elderberry blossom tea makes a good eye-wash to cure pink eye (—Mrs. David Miller).

Pleurisy: Put 1 tblsp. of turpentine in a quart of hot water. Soak woolen cloths in this solution and apply as hot as possible to the sore chest. Cover with a plastic cloth. Repeat as necessary. Also 1 or 2 capsules cayenne takes away the pain. Repeat as needed, but not on an empty stomach!

Pneumonia: Here are two Amish salves for pneumonia. Weaver's salve: Take ½ lb. of vaseline, 2 oz. gum camphor, 1 oz. turpentine, ½ tsp. carbolic acid, and beeswax the size of a walnut. Melt together and stir. Here's another one: melt

6 oz. lard, add 2 oz. camphor pulverized and 3 oz. beeswax, as it melts slowly. Then add 3 oz. of white rosin, and 2 oz. red balsam of Peru, with 2 drams of oil of cedar. Stir often as it is melting. After it's done, stir in 2 oz. of turpentine while cooling. Store in a covered tin or jar. When applying this, spread it on a wax paper, put it on the chest, cover with a cloth and pin fast to the shirt or dress. Keep it on until the patient can't tolerate any more. Later rub off the chest with alcohol to keep it from being itchy. This salve will also remove moles with frequent application.

Here is another poultice for pneumonia. Mix flaxseed meal and black mustard (ground) in equal parts and apply to the chest. Keep covered. Patient should drink hot pennyroyal tea.

Sinus: A bad sinus infection was healed by repeatedly putting a pinch of golden seal on the tongue (—Willy Beiler). Another good sinus remedy is to drink golden seal tea, while eliminating all milk products from your diet. You may even sniff (snuff) golden seal powder to clear the sinus! Here is another remedy: in the evening, take ¼ tsp. of salt in a cup and draw it up through the nose and down through the mouth; gargle with the salt water. Or, take ¼ tsp. of baking soda in a cup of warm water and drink it in the evening before going to bed. Olba's Inhalers helps.

Sinus infection: Soak a handful of pennyroyal leaves in 6 oz. of sweet almond oil until the oil turns green; then add a few grams of horehound powder; use a few drops of this in the nose for immediate decongestion.

Strep throat: Apply a poultice of grated garden beets on the outside of the throat. They will turn a greenish color. Continue renewing the beet poultice until beets do not discolor. Also, suck garlic cloves. Take red clover tops drops. 2,000 mg. vitamin C powder 2 or 3 times daily fights most any infections!

Styes: Wash with warm chamomile tea.

Swollen glands: Gargle with a mixture made from 7 lime rinds boiled in milk. Another good gargle for this is made from rue cooked in milk. Also, you may apply flannel soaked in apple cider vinegar, warm. Do not ever squeeze the glands! Congestion should gradually disappear. A good herbal combination is: Mullein and Lobelia.

Tonsillitis: Gargle with red clover tops tea. Externally, apply a poultice of onions. Do not allow the tonsils to be removed except as a desperate measure of last resort. There is a purpose for them. A Glandular Thymus helps fight off infection. A good herbal tincture contains: Scullcap, Lobelia, Valerian Root, Myrrh Gum, Black Cohosh and Cayenne. It is a good anti-spasmodic and nerve tincture also.

Toothaches: Soak cotton in clove oil and place it next to the aching tooth. Or cut a fig in half, lengthwise, and lay it against the aching tooth. Also take bone meal tablets. Taking a herbal combination of Horsetail Grass, Comfrey Root, Oat Straw and Lobelia helps.

One Amish woman said a herbal combination of Horsetail Grass, Comfrey Root, Oat Straw and Lobelia taken in capsule form taken regularly stopped their visits to the dentist.

Whooping cough: Make a tea by boiling 1 tsp. of wild cherry bark and 1 tblsp. red sage in a pint of water. Take 1 tsp. five times daily.

Another **whooping cough** remedy: steep ½ tsp. dried, crushed green peach tree leaves, in 1 quart boiling water for 10 minutes. Take 1 tblsp. of this tea every hour, with a few drops of honey.

Another **whooping cough** remedy: Take 3-4 chestnut leaves and add to a pint of boiling water. Steep to make a tea, sweeten with honey and let children drink of it 5 or 6 times daily.

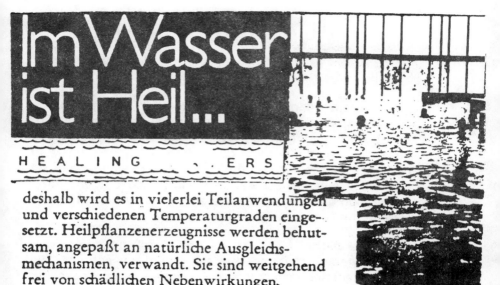

Im Wasser ist Heil...

deshalb wird es in vielerlei Teilanwendungen
und verschiedenen Temperaturgraden einge-
setzt. Heilpflanzenerzeugnisse werden behut-
sam, angepaßt an natürliche Ausgleichs-
mechanismen, verwandt. Sie sind weitgehend
frei von schädlichen Nebenwirkungen.

Chapter 7: *Recipes for Skin and Eliminatory System*

We might subtitle this chapter, the Water of Life. It is
primarily concerned with cleanliness within and without.
Water is the greatest cleansing medium. Dr. Simon Baruch
once listed 12 uses of water in medicine:

1. As a stimulant (a glass given to a person feeling faint); 2.
A sedative (a glass of hot water before retiring); 3. A tonic (a
glass of mineral water to refresh your blood); 4. A diuretic
(copious water drinking flushes the kidneys); 5. A
diaphoretic (hot water, drunk or bathed in, can induce
sweating); 6. An emetic (lukewarm water can cause
vomiting); 7. A purgative (warm water on rising can help
bowel movements); 8. A promoter of better metabolism
(more frequent drinking favors alteration); 9. An antiseptic
(washing a wound with water can prevent infection); 10. An
antipyretic (bathing the brow and body can reduce fever);
11. An hypnotic (staring at rhythmically running water or

ripples can induce a trance); 12. A local anesthetic (cool water on a burn kills pain). So we must absolutely say, "Thank God for *water!*"

Don't underestimate the aesthetic worth of water. If you can, build your house where you can see and hear a river or spring with running water. We have a little spring below our house, and we dug a small pond into which it can trickle. It refreshes the eye and soothes the nerves. Having renounced electricity, many Amish set up a water wheel or some other application of water power. Water is a favorite Amish drink. Garden mint tea is another favorite.

Medicinal baths: Many of the first Greek hospitals were healing "temples" founded at the site of hot springs. The curative regimen included fasting, dieting, herbs, massage, counselling, rest, and exercise. The ancients had the proverb that the three best doctors are "Dr. Diet, Dr. Quiet and Dr. Happiness."

Patients were bathed in hot springs water, cold water, sea water, given mud baths, steam baths, and even sea-shore sand baths. So valued were *hot springs* as curative centers, the Bible gives one man's name as "the boy who discovered a *hot springs* in the wasteland while he was grazing his father's donkeys!" (Genesis 36:24).

The ancient town beside the Sea of Galilee we now know as Tiberias was originally called *Chamath* ["hot springs"]. Later the Romans built bathing establishments there, then the Turks, and today the state of Israel maintains a modern hydrotherapy ("water cure") institute there. I had the privilege of bathing there and also at the hot sulphur springs beside the Dead Sea, at En-Gedi. The baths at En-Gedi were near where the Essenes maintained their community, origin of the Dead Sea Scrolls. They devoted their lives to copying the Word of God, living simply and peacably, and restricting themselves to a life of quietness and holiness like some ancient sect of Amish.

Many ancient peoples seemed to have believed that "cleanliness is next to godliness." I have had the privilege of visiting many hot springs used by the Indians in the south-western U.S., Mexico, Guatemala and Costa Rica. It is a soothing and relaxing experience to soak or swim in such springs and pools. The Amish are also fond of going to such places. Probably it is the heat of the water plus the dissolved minerals in the water which is curative.

Bath therapy was sometimes called balneotherapy, or more generally *hydrotherapy.* The constant bathing in as well as drinking of the water, kept the bowels and kidneys active and the pores of the skin open. These are the principal channels for eliminating body wastes and poisons. Each square inch of our skin has 3,500 sweat tubes or perspiration outlets. Altogether there are almost 40 miles of these drain tiles in our skin. No wonder the skin has been called our greatest organ of elimination! To block these drains would lead to death, as has been discovered when people were painted in such a way that their pores were closed; they strangled in toxins.

Many a modern American who sprays himself with colognes and deoderants to prevent sweating, would be horrified to realize that his body needs to sweat to eliminate toxins! We don't have to smell sweaty but we do have to perspire toxins out of our systems or risk illness. I try to get up a good sweat each day. If your work does not require much physical effort, you can take a hot shower to help your skin eliminate toxins. The ailments that follow, in one way or another, are the results of toxins that need to be eliminated, or injuries to the skin. Zinc Lozenges from Zinc Orotate-Aspartate taken daily has reduced my body odors and colds. (S. Chupp)

Acne: Taking 3 activated charcoal tablets, 3 times daily before meals, will improve three fourths of all acne conditions. Also avoid *all* chocolate. A good herbal combination is Dandelion Root, Sarsaparilla Root, Burdock

Root, Licorice Root, Echinacea, Yellow Dock Root, Kelp, Cayenne, and Chaparral.

Another remedy for *acne* is to keep the facial pores clean by occasional facial steam baths. You can lean carefully over a steaming pan of hot water, with a towel funnelling the steam to your face. Many skin eruptions are also due to vitamin B complex deficiency.

Athlete's foot: This fungus infection of the skin is killed by applying the raw juice of Jewelweed (Touch-me-not plant). Another remedy is to mix sulphur, powdered egg shell and iodine with lard and apply as salve. Of some 73 plants that were tested for fungicidal properties, the most powerful were Jewelweed, Nasturtium, and Muskmelon! Many Amish wash their feet daily in Boric Acid water to eliminate odors and athlete's foot. They also sprinkle the Boric Acid powder in socks and shoes.

Baths: If you are unable to visit a hot springs, make your own hydrotherapy at home by making a strong tea from any of the following herbs and adding it to your hot bath water before you take a relaxing soak! —rose petals, mint leaves, sweet marjoram, lemon balm, verbena, lavender. We happen to have a whirlpool bath in our house. I like to get a packet of spa minerals and add them to the whirlpool before I get in. It is most refreshing! (Do not stay longer than 15 minutes as it can weaken you. Some people foolish enough to drink wine and laze around in the hot tubs too long have become unconscious and drowned.) If you do not happen to be near a health food store where you can buy the spa minerals in a packet, a cup of plain epsom salts in your tub will serve as a detoxifying soak. Add 2 tblsp. of dry mustard for aching muscles. A solution of bicarbonate of soda in the bath water **kills perspiration odors.**

Bee stings: If a bumble bee ever stings you, you will want to mix equal parts of soda and vinegar to make a paste to put on it. If you don't have those ingredients handy, apply a fresh cut onion to draw poison.

Burns: The simplest remedy is to apply cool water to relieve pain. Burns that are over wide areas need immediate medical attention. Smaller burns can also be relieved by applying fresh aloe vera gel; break a branch off the aloe vera plant and squeeze some of the gel gently onto the burn. Or, puncture a vitamin E capsule and drop the oil onto the burn. This heals it quickly and prevents a scar from forming. Old timers melted lard and stirred in cattail fuzz, to make a thick paste to put on burns. Some Amish put honey on small burns. They also spray deluted Willard water on burns to prevent scarring, etc.

Other remedies for **burns:** Make a paste of one part lard to one part flour and apply to small burns. Also apple butter is pretty good to put on burns. A tea is made from cheese plant (the common mallow) and cooled, then swabbed on burns. (This is also good for infections that will not heal.)

Blood in the urine: A two-year old boy, ill with urinary tract infection, had blood in his urine, was being dosed to no avail by the doctors with strong antibiotics; instead of hospitalizing him as the doctors advised, the parents took him to an Amish herb lady who gave him horsetail grass tea and he was cured at once. Comfrey Root tea is also helpful.

Boils: Isaiah's prescription of a mashed fig poultice is used (II Kings 20:7). Salt baths are also used (Ezekiel 16:4).

Bleeding badly: Of course, one should try to apply pressure at the proper pressure points to stop bleeding, or even put a tourniquet on (being careful to loosen it occasionally so as not to cut off all circulation). But the Amish in pioneer times also used a certain Scripture verse, quoting and claiming it by faith, to stop bleeding (Ezekiel 16:6). Thus it required faith for healing.

Black heads: Use soap and water, lathering freely; dry, rinse thoroughly, then squeeze or press out the larger black heads with the fingers. Afterwards sponge with witch hazel daily.

Bleeding cuts: Cover the cut with unglazed brown paper wet with vinegar. Also Cayenne will stop bleeding on cuts and internally.

Burns: Some dip a burn in cold fresh cream, if available.

Bruises: The Amish use a "zeek schmeer" made of ½ lb. fresh lard, 3 oz. white rosin, 2 drams balsam of Peru, ¼ lb. beeswax, and 2 oz. pulverized camphor. Putting all these ingredients together, melt slowly over low heat (it takes most of a day). Then take from stove and add 1 oz. turpentine; mix well and store in baby food jars. Combats infection, heals wounds. Also it is used for sore cow teats.

Cancer of skin: Oxalis (wood sorrel) leaves are crushed into a pulp and applied as a poultice; is said to pull out the core of the cancer, and hurts, but heals. Old Molly Meeks is said to have cured many skin cancers by applying a paste of honey mixed with arsenic, then covering it with beef suet; apply and remove for three days in succession (but frankly, this sounds risky to us). Others also report the use of powdered arsenic mixed with enough honey to make a paste. The Irish used to use ground ivy herb, a low, creeping plant; they would make a strong tea of it and drink it for cancer. A safer remedy is Aveloz or Pau d' Arco Ointment. The *Original* Purple Flowering *Pau d' Arco* (Ipe Roxo) is available from Health Stores, imported from A.S. Grozdea Co. in Brazil.

Cancer in general: This dread disease kills one out of four Americans. However, Amish herb users are known to have some success in using two South American herbs for cancer, tumors and cysts in general. One is Pau d' Arco tea, drunk as a blood cleanser and general tonic. In Brazil it is also called *Ipe Roxo* or *Taheebo* and was used for centuries by the Indians. Dr. Walter Accorsi of Sao Paulo experimented with this herb and found it useful in eliminating pain and multiplying red corpuscles in cancer victims. In Brazil, the purple flowering is the best one. The Indians boil the bark slowly for 10 minutes, then steep it 10

.more minutes keeping it covered. They put 1 tsp. per cup of tea and drink one cup 3 to 6 times throughout the day. The Indians find that adding 5 drops Aveloz (another herbal tea) in Pau d' Arco tea helps but this is taken only 3 times a day. Many testimonials say: It helped high blood pressure, headaches, prostate, nerves, tonic, sleep better, helps constipation, digestion pain, heart, sugar count, cystic fibrosis and menstrual problems, bleeding, kidneys, varicose veins, etc. But some say they had just a little effect. Of course, tobacco and alcohol works against most herbs. Don't use metal pots! Use *glass* or *porcelain*.

Cataracts: Mrs. Katie Layman kept from having a cataract operation by just bathing her eyes in warm salt water, followed by warm vinegar water, several times a day. The doctor who had diagnosed cataracts was amazed to examine her later and said, "Why, the Lord gave you your second eye sight!" One woman in Middlebury said she could see better after spraying a catalyst altered water in her eyes. It took some time.

Canker sores in mouth: Use sage tea for mouth sores (or sore eyes). Or, apply a pinch of powdered sage against the sore. Or, apply golden seal powder, or raw onion.

Chapped lips: Use lanolin lotion.

Corns: Soak your feet in warm water for about 15 minutes; then cut a small piece of lemon peel and place the inside of it against the corn, tying it on, and let it stay there all night. Do this for three nights and the corn should lift out. You can also buy *Men-Zo-Lin* at Health Food Stores.

Dandruff: Secure a small amount of pure coconut oil; rub this in your hair for a few days and dandruff should disappear. Burdock and sage tea can be used as a rinse.

Dental pain: Of couse see your dentist for repairs, but meanwhile eat asparagus every day (fresh or canned) and you will be able to bear the pain. [—from John Hartman].

Diaper rash: We have found that vitamin A and D ointment is the best remedy! Be sure to dry the diapers in the sunlight after washing them. Some use cornstarch also. One Amish woman said that sulphur pine tar works wonders!

Diuretic for kidney stones: Use cucumber juice; or tea from ½ avocado leaf. Or take brown corn seed, 3 teaspoonfuls, and put in a pint of water; allow to steep, then drink one cup daily. This is said to be good also for gall stones.

Dry skin: Mix together one part each of cocoa butter, glycerine, lanolin, rosewater and elderflower water. Apply to the skin daily.

Eczema: Make a salve by combining one lb. of butter (without salt), 2 oz. of red precipitate (fulminate of mercury), and 4 oz. of venus turpentine; stir well and pour water off. Use once daily in evening, applying lightly so as not to blister the skin; repeat for three days. [This sounds risky to us; beware.] Here is a remedy that sounds safer to me: For *eczema,* gather black poplar buds (Balm of Gilead) in the spring, when they are sticky, before the frost is fully gone; then boil them in olive oil, strain and make a salve; apply regularly. A safe natural herbal combination is: Barberry, Wild Yam, Cramp Bark, Fennel Seed, Ginger, Catnip and Peppermint. Take capsules 15 minutes before meals.

Felon: To cure a felon on a finger, heat turpentine as hot as you can stand it, then plunge your finger into it[!]; or, plunge the finger with the felon on it into hot tomato juice! Or, plunge finger into hot water, again and again. Or, take the inside film from an egg shell, and apply it to draw felon.

Face, white spots on, also on neck: Make a salve of hog lard, limes and sulphur and paint it on the spots. Keep applying until they disappear.

Festering skin cancers: Apply green flesh of the Pipe Organ cactus as a poultice. Also effective for skin cancer is to take a small green papaya (about a pound in weight), grate one third of it each night and bind it on with rags and a big sock or plastic sack on top. This has also been used to treat infected athlete's foot.

Grandma Hofer's Salve: For sores and boils, drawing out poison and slivers; take ½ cup of beeswax cut fine, and 1 cup of lard (½ goose fat if possible), add to these one well-rounded teaspoon of powdered resin; melt slowly on the stove, stirring constantly until melted together. Remove to cool, stirring constantly until thick and smooth.

Hand lotion: A Hutterite recipe from Alberta, Canada; take 4 oz. glycerine, 4 oz. alcohol, and 1 oz. quince seed; pour one pint of boiling soft water on the quince seed, let it soak overnight, then strain and add the other ingredients. (If too thick, add water).

Freckles: Bathe the face in fresh buttermilk; or, mix 2 oz. of sour milk with 2 drams grated horseradish and 6 drams of cornmeal; spread this mixture between thin muslin and apply to the affected parts at night, leaving on as long as possible (but be careful not to get it in the eyes).

Another treatment for *freckles,* which sounds like a superstition, is to wash your face in the morning dew, while going barefoot!

Enemas: In recent years some Amish have been using coffee enemas. At least that is a better use for coffee than drinking it! Personally, I would not use it at either end! Aloe Vera juice enemas are used with good success.

Hand lotion: Here is another good recipe for this; mix equal parts of bay rum and glycerine, and mix well; apply to rough hands.

Hair care: Shampoo the hair with your own formula and avoid harsh chemical detergents and chemical dyes. Our old-timers used to use rosemary leaves, camomile flowers, rosewater, and very mild home-made soap (or Indian soap plant bulb, when they could find it). A beaten egg was added to the shampoo and natural coconut oil. All this made for softer, more glossy, less tangled hair. Rinse well after shampooing. For **baldness** and premature loss of natural hair color, take red clover tops liquid extract, 40 drops daily. Use vinegar as a rinse with sage tea added to it.

Insect bites: Take 2 oz. olive oil, add 1 dram of carbolic acid, 1 dram pennyroyal oil, 1 dram of cedar oil, 2 drams of citronella oil, 2 drams of tincture of camphor, ½ dram of acetic acid; mix well. By applying on exposed parts will ward off insects and applied to bites it destroys the poison and heals the soreness. (—from Mrs. Cornelius E. Miller).

Mosquito bite relief: Moisten a bar of soap and rub on the bite; it will stop itching and the soap acts as a disinfectant. To keep flies and mosquitoes off rub citronella on skin. Works for pets, too. EX-NOLO-Thylene applied on bite will work wonders in minutes.

Pimples: Dry them with lard and flour paste (equal parts, applied to draw). See *eczema* (herbal formula).

Poison ivy: Bathing the affected parts in sassafras tea should banish it. Or, bruise and crush some stems and leaves of the plant called Jewelweed (or Touch-me-not). One application of this juice does more good than a pint of calamine lotion! Washing with Tansy tea is also a good treatment for poison ivy. Exnolothylene can be bought in health stores. It gets rid of it in 2-3 days!

Prickly heat: This affliction can make babies miserable; one soothing relief for them is to gently rub the affected parts with a watermelon rind. Or, sponge with equal parts of vinegar and water, then dry the skin and powder with one part boric acid and one part corn starch (**Caution!** Keep all boric acid away from baby's mouth; it is **poisonous!**).

Scar tissue: Repeatedly rub cocoa butter on scar tissue;

gradually it will go away if not too old. Or, for any cuts or blemishes or any skin disease that may leave a scar; rub castor oil on it a few times a day for several weeks; it will usually cause the scar to vanish (—David E. Yoder). Vitamin E oil rubbed on daily also helps.

Sunburn lotion: One of the best is aloe vera gel; break a leaf off the plant and slice it in half lengthwise; the inner sticky gel is very healing for sunburn.

Warts: Use celandine juice on warts; use milkweed juice on them; castor oil rubbed on them often causes them to dry up. Or, wash in water to which a quantity of washing soda has been added. Let your hand dry without wiping; repeat until warts dissolve. Aveloz or Black ointment works good.

How I Collected this Amish Formulary:

This present book was the fruit of 12 years of collecting Amish Folk remedy formulas. Many of these I gathered from readers of my weekly column in *The Sugarcreek Budget.* For years I wrote a health column for that newspaper, widely read among the Amish. I requested readers to send me any good recipes they wanted to share with the public through this book. Others I found in old journals, papers, or by interviews with Amish herbalists. As far as I know, this is the only Amish formulary ever published. Here are some of the collected samples:

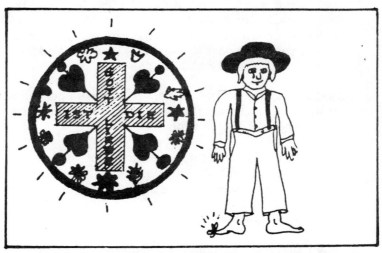

Chapter 8: **Recipes for Nervous System and Personality**

We might subtitle this chapter "the Word of life." Long ago the Bible pointed out the close connection between emotional health and physical health: *"A merry heart doeth good like a medicine: but a broken spirit drieth the bones."* (Proverbs 17:22). In this chapter we shall list some of the healthy attitudes that the Amish use to overcome emotional sickness.

In the picture above, I have drawn an Amish boy with an injured toe. Beside him is a hearts-and-flowers symbol with the cross inscribed "Gott ist die Liebe" ("God is love" in German). The poem on page 14 pointed out that "Mother love" is by far one of the best ingredients of all old-timey remedies. Every physical hurt can wound the spirit, so whoever tended the injured toe of the boy in the picture, she likely also wisely soothed his hurt feelings!

Instead of living in an impersonal universe 'evolving' from some primordial 'Big Bang,' Amish live in a universe created by God-Who-Is-Love. That faith-confidence overcomes a host of fears which torment and bedevil their more skeptical fellowcitizens. The guide book of the Amish is the Bible, the *Word of life.* We believe it contains the secrets of **happiness**. This book of health recipes would be incomplete without sharing with you some Amish wit and wisdom based on Biblical truths.

One of the favorite Amish songs is entitled "Gott Ist Die Liebe" (God Is Love). Here is a rough translation of some of the verses: "God is Love! He let me be saved; God is love, He loves even me! Thou healest, O Love, all my troubles; Thou calmest, O Love, my deepest woe!" And that's the way it is folks: God loves even *YOU!*Give Him a chance to prove it by opening your heart to Him!

Adversity: The Bible says, "A brother is born for adversity" (Prov. 17:17). That is why we don't need insurance companies; the church is our family and if my barn burns down, my brothers will help me build another one.

Accidents: What men too easily call "accidents" are not occasions for blame and guilt. They are to be accepted as part of God's "providence," and an opportunity to help one another. "All things work together for good to them that love God." (Romans 8:28).

Affliction: Often leads us closer to God and to one another (Psalms 119:67). Which of us has suffered unjustly, as Jesus did? What if we had to suffer or even die for our faith? Better to be killed than to kill others; martyrs go to heaven; murderers go to hell.

Alms: Whatever we give away in this life, without claiming, boasting or publicizing it, that is treasure we are laying up in heaven! (Matthew 6:3, Mark 10:21).

Anger: Grievous words stir up anger (Prov. 15:1) but a soft answer turns away wrath (Prov. 15:1). Don't let the sun go down on your anger.(Eph. 4:26). Settle quarrels quickly or they will settle you! To hold a grudge or burn with resentment will eat you up like a cancer! Forgive others so you may be forgiven.(Mt. 6:12-15).

Baptism: When you are baptised, it is a covenant with God and the church. That is why a baby cannot be truly baptised. It is a pledge before witnesses to be faithful to Christ and His church.

Blessings: Blessings are the gifts of God which make us happy. The greatest gift is God's Son; if we have Jesus, we have the hidden manna we need for every circumstance.

A happy man is one who counts the blessings he has, rather than the things he doesn't have. When we are counting blessings, let's start with all the wonderful gifts of nature we get free. Consider the *sun,* for example. Sunlight turns our tomatoes and strawberries red, ripens our wheat to a shimmering gold, warms our houses through solar heat, firewood, and coal (which are all forms of sunlight energy). Fresh air and sunlight cure our sniffles and sunlight vitamins prevent rickets. Even the small baby born with jaundice is best healed in bright sunlight. Thank God for the sun!

> We read of numerous powders and pills,
> Miraculous healing for all our ills,
> But rarely can we find in one
> The healing we get *free* from the sun!

Curses: If someone curses you, bless them, and it will transform their curse! Overcome evil with good (Romans 12:21) or evil will overcome you. If your enemy is hungry, feed him, and melt his fury with gentleness. (Rom. 12:20). A man whose speech is full of damning and cursing is a man who is in rebellion against his Maker. Those who take God's name in vain will not go unpunished (Exodus 20:7). Besides, cursing and swearing just prove you have a poor vocabulary.

Conscience: A clear conscience is the best pillow. A

conscience enlightened by the Word of God is a safe guide, but not conscience alone. Many will join in with a crowd to shed blood but a truly conscientious man will refuse to hurt a fellow human being. If the Bible constrains our conscience, and not the nation, we shall be conscientious objectors to any kind of war. (Mt. 5:21-48, I Peter 2:19-25, 3:9-14).

Contentment: The first Amish bishop who came to America (in 1749), Jacob Hertzler, named his pioneer homestead **Contentment.** Behind him in Europe were wars and persecutions. Facing him in America were Indian raids and revolution. But to those who cried out that he must flee, he simply echoed the words of the apostle Paul: "I have learned in whatsoever state I am, therewith to be *content."* (Phil. 4:11).

Ever since then, it has been the goal of the Amish life style to cultivate contentment. This is a Biblical goal. "Better is a handful with quietness, than both the hands full with travail and vexation of spirit." (Eccles. 4:6). 'And having food and raiment let us be therewith *content."* (I Tim. 6:8). "But godliness with *contentment* is great gain." (1 Tim 6:6).

If the beauty of the home is order, the blessing of the home is *contentment.* He that is *content* has enough; he that complains has too much. Lucretius said, The greatest wealth is to live content with little, for there is never want where the mind is satisfied." *Contentment* is more than a kingdom! If we seek first the kingdom of God, then everything else that is necessary will be supplied.

Death: Amish do not buy the fancy American way of death, with exorbitant funerals and expensive caskets. The brothers make the casket of pine or oak, the grave is dug by them, too. The planting of the corpse is a simple affair, without ostentatious display. They do not need to prove that they loved the deceased. They bury the remains with simplicity and good taste and are convinced the deceased has himself departed to a better world. Buying expensive caskets and cosmetic jobs and flower displays is for those who are guilty about something and are trying to prove they "really loved him." The Amishman says, Show me love while I am living instead of trying to convince the undertaker.

Depression: Everyone at some time in life is faced with a feeling of defeat or depression. A born-again Amishman will again have the advantage here because he believes what the Bible says: "Nay, in all these things, we are more than conquerors through Him that loved us!" (Rom. 8:37). Wise Amish women know that there is such a thing as a post-partum depression possible after birth, so they take extra vitamin B complex and Red Clover tops liquid extract to calm and replenish the depleted nerves. The best prescription for depression is count your many blessings!

Divorce: An Amish Mennonite minister was once asked by some Protestant ministers, "We understand that your church does not allow divorces. Don't you have a lot of unhappy marriages?" He replied, "Some, but not nearly as many as where they allow divorces!" In fact, Jesus also lived in a time when divorce was made legally easy. He insisted on restoring the permanency of marriage and stated that divorce would be impossible without people hardening their hearts to one another! Mt. 19:3-12). Divorce is practically unknown among the Amish and marriage problems are worked out by reconciliation and counselling. Preventing broken homes is better than trying to decide to do something with the pieces afterwards!

Diseases (terminal): Cancer is a major cause of death in industrialized countries. A Swiss physician, Dr. Walter Blumer, reports that he had 75 patients that had died of cancer in a twelve-year period. 72 of them lived within fifty yards of the highway! More of his patients that lived close to highways had headaches, sleep disorders, nervousness and digestive upsets, than people living farther away. The pollutants from passing traffic and stress of the traffic, are a contributing factor to many terminal diseases. If we get out of the "fast lane" of life, and retire more into the pure atmosphere of rural living, we shall live better and *longer!*

Dealing with pests: Cucumber peelings left around the floors will usually drive cockroaches out. Powdered cinnamon (or powdered cayenne pepper) spread around the edges of the kitchen will usually drive ants away.

The Amish are a people who value their privacy. One of the great nuisances to them is the horde of tourists who sometimes invade their communities to stare at them. Normally courteous to strangers, they can be provoked to sharp replies. One Amishman was pointed at by an obese tourist lady who said: "Look at that odd man!" Returning her look, he saw her paint, powder, artificial hairstyle, gaudy clothes and bulging shorts, and could not resist replying: "It wonders me **who** is **really** the **ODD ONE!**" Another tourist is reported to have said to an Amishman, I "I once grew a beard like yours, but when I saw how terrible I looked, I shaved it off!" The Amishman cooly replied: "I used to have a face like yours, too, and when I saw how terrible it looked, I grew a beard!"

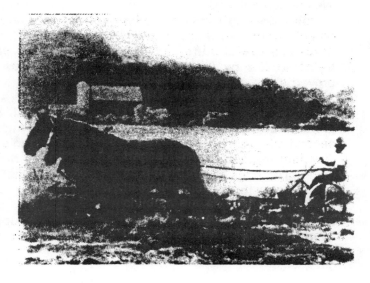

Another story is told of two men sitting in a bus station in Reading, Pennsylvania. One was a bearded Amishman, the other a very old man. The old man, seeing his bus coming, painfully stood up and said to the Amishman, "I am suffering from arthritis." "Well, I am glad to meet you," said the Amishman, "I am Stoltzfus from New Holland."

Because the Bible says, "a merry heart doeth good like a medicine," the Amish appreciate humor. One Amishman replied to a man who splashed mortar on him and asked if he was hurt: "No, I'm just mortified!"

Devil: The Bible says, "Resist the devil and he will flee from you." (James 4:7). American teenagers are fond of wearing "Tee" shirts with the legend, "The devil made me do it." The Amish believe that is a "cop out" or attempt to escape responsibility for one's actions. If you yield to temptation, it is your fault! A favorite Amish proverb is "idleness is the devil's workshop."

Diligence in work: To the Amish one of the greatest sins in the catalogue is **Laziness.** The Bible says: "Seest thou a man diligent in his business? he shall stand before kings." We are admonished to be "not slothful in business; fervent in spirit; serving the Lord." (Romans 12:11). Every Amish parent wants to have his children be hard workers, producing useful fruits of labor, instead of lazy parasites trying to live by their wits while loafing. A few Amish proverbs about good workers:

An Industrious wife is the best savings account. A loafer prefers hurting himself carrying a heavy load, to making a second trip. A loafer lives by stealing other men's labors. "Let him that stole steal no more: but rather let him labor, working with his hands the thing which is good, that he may have to give to him that needeth." (Eph. 4:28).

Dumb Dutch? Many stories are told about the supposedly "dumb Dutch." What appears to the public to be "dumb" may often be a kind of a shrewd peasant logic. An Amish proverb says, "We get too soon old, and too late smart." An Amish boy tried to explain the backwardness of his brother to the teacher by saying, "It ain't he can't learn, it's just he doesn't remember anything he learn." A tourist complained about the chicken being tough in a Dutch restaurant and the Dutch waitress replied: "It's tougher when there's none."

A group of school boys tried to scare little Amos, an Amish boy. They jumped out at him with an imitation skeleton. He didn't bat an eyelash so they asked, "Aren't you afraid of spooks and skeletons?" Amos replied, "Why, there ain't no such thing as a ghost, and a skeleton is nothing but a stack of bones with the people scraped off."

While some Amish are gullible, as in any group of people, most are quite shrewd enough not to panic like many of their English neighbors. Watching a parade of protestors against nuclear war, an Amishman was asked "Aren't you afraid of the Third World War?" He replied, "The Bible says there will be wars and rumors of wars until the End, then Jesus will come. Only a fool would fear the wars and not fear God Who will judge all mankind."

Education: While many Americans labor under the delusion that a man cannot be a success without a college education, the Amish are more concerned to prepare their children for useful lives by a good basic education and learning a trade (farming, carpentry, masonry, cabinet making, plumbing). It is notorious that many city schools turn out children who cannot even read. Standard achievement tests given to the pupils in Amish and Mennonite parochial schools have proven that their general scores are high above the national average. Rather than push their children into higher education, in an economy where many college graduates are unemployed, the Amish prefer to produce handcraftsmen who build houses and farms.

Envy: If a man does not envy the lot of others but is content with his own lifestyle, he is not easily moved by high-powered advertising. An Amishman just laughs at advertising which tries to get him to buy designer jeans, sports cars, and other fashionable status symbols.

What our general society calls "ambition" and "success" is often just people running in the rat race to keep ahead of their neighbors. Is the happy man one who has money to buy things he does not need, to impress people he does not like, or is he the man who does not *want* more than he *needs*?

The Amish are curious about **television, rock music, radios** and the drug culture, but they avoid all these things because they see the results are crime, juvenile delinquency, divorce, nervous breakdowns and social disorders. An Amishman was asked if he did not miss radio and television. He replied, "They are selling something I don't need: entertainment, multiplying your wants for things you don't need, and discontentment. It is not so much what you eat that makes you sick, but what *is eating you* because of what you are looking at and listening to. I don't envy you. I pity you."

Family: One of the greatest Amish strengths is their strong love of family. The Dutch word *Freundschaft* means their extended family of relatives. A lot of time is spent in visiting the *Freundschaft.* An Amishman cut off from his relatives would be lonely indeed, unlike the modern urban dweller who lives in atomistic isolation (and often in alienation to others as well as to his environment). Close-knit families are the rule instead of the generation gap and disrespect for older people.

One of the mad, sad things about modern urban society is it's trying to be a "youth culture." Middle aged and older people dye their hair and paint their lips and diet and wear "mod" clothes to try to appear young. The Amishman accepts the cycles of nature, welcomes middle age and cherishes old age. They shun abortion as well as "mercy killing of the aged." Each member of the family is made to feel useful and wanted. Grandparents are not warehoused in institutions but kept at home in their own cottage on the farm (called the "Dawdy Haus"). Every child should have the privilege of growing up in an extended family. It gives him both respect and the confidence of a secure old age. The Amish spurn social security, welfare, government hand-outs, crop insurances, and such. A favorite Scripture for them is: "But if any provide not for his own, and specially for those of his own house, he hath denied the faith, and is worse than an infidel." (I Timothy 5:8).

In our modern industrial society, it is not unheard of for the governor of Colorado to have recently announced: "[Elderly people who are terminally ill have a] duty to die and get out of the way. Let the other society, our kids, build a reasonable life." But the Bible does not speak of dealing "death with dignity" to the aged and ill. Instead it speaks of the *dignity of old age*: "The hoary head is a crown of glory." (Proverbs 16:31). "The glory of young men is their strength: and the beauty of old men is the gray head." (Proverbs 20:29). "Children's children are the crown of old men; and the glory of children are their fathers." (Prov. 17:6). Only a sick society despises the elderly. After all, in the course of nature *we* are growing older. If we reject the aged, the next generation will reject us. What a man sows, he reaps.

Fear: The Bible gives the Amish standard here, "The Lord is my light and my salvation; whom shall I fear? the Lord is the strength of my life; of whom shall I be afraid?" (Read Psalm 27:1). The secret is: "There is no fear in love, but perfect love casteth out fear." (I John 4:18). In colonial days, there was a very strong Amish miller named Strong Jacob Yoder. He could carry two 200 pound sacks of wheat at one time. One day a famous wrestler came to his mill to challenge him to a wrestling match. Strong Jacob refused to fight the man. After all, God had given him his strength not to fight men but to do useful work. But the stranger kept insisting on a fight and finally attacked Strong Jacob. Regretfully, Jacob grabbed him like one would a child, tucked him under his arm and with his other arm grabbed a 200 pound sack of wheat and carried both up the stairs and into the mill store house, depostiting both the would-be wrestler and the sack of wheat!

Group Self-hatred: A strange psychological illness first observed by social psychologists among socially mobile Orthodox Jews. Some who had been raised in strict orthodox tradition, to speak Yiddish. wear modest clothing, and keep the observances of Judaism, when they got older would leave the group, shun any observances and customs that set them apart from modern urban society, and despised their upbringing. Some ex-Amish are found with these same resentments. It seems to come from replacing the in-group ideals with the ideals and goals of the fashionable society. Some such Amish join more liberal Protestant churches or even try to become completely assimilated socialites. But how can a man deny his heritage and be happy? If you are always running away from your background, you are chained to it by reaction and resentment.

Happiness: "Happy is the man that findeth wisdom; . . . Her ways are ways of pleasantness and all her paths are peace." (Prov. 3:13/17). Happiness is a healthy outlook on life. If you cannot change your circumstances, you can change yourself to adapt to those circumstances. There is a proverb, "If you want to be the picture of health, keep in a good frame of mind." Bible believers believe that happiness cannot be separated from holiness and godliness. An Amishman is for this reason very devoted to the practice of *separation* from pride, anger, malice, lust, greed, fashion and vanity.

Holidays: Great workers like the Amish cherish their holidays. They do only the most necessary chores for their animals on the Lord's Day. Good Friday is observed in remembrance of Christ's sacrifice on the cross to redeem mankind. Ascension Day is observed to commemorate Christ ascending to heaven and His making intercession there for those who pray to Him. A curious Amish notion is

84

that Ascension Day is the time to gather medicinal plants.

Those who collected such medicinal plants often gathered them in three's such as, three plants from the woods (elder blossoms, wintergreen, dogwood flowers); three plants from the garden (horehound, thyme, sage); three plants from the field (catnip, ground ivy, cinquefoil).

Amish observe Easter, of course, and Christmas, and even some observe Old Christmas (January 6). Besides, they have certain superstitions or notions about some other holidays (or perhaps there is some wisdom in calculating that we don't know about): No gardening or planting should be done between Good Friday and Easter. The best time to sow clover is on St. Patrick's Day. Also, there are certain recommended days to mow thistles. I used to think that was a superstition until it was explained to me that it usually rained after those mowing days and rainwater entered the thistle stalks and rotted them so that they would not regrow!

Holy kiss: One of the Amish practices based on the New Testament, where brother greets brother with a holy kiss, and sister greets sister (this is only between members of the same sexes). It is another sign of the family closeness of the church. Where love has cooled off, this ordinance tends to be neglected. Psychologists tell us that one of the problems of our sick urban society is that so many people are starved for affection. Physical affection is often shown among the Amish; this helps give security and acceptance.

Hostility and the heart: Recent studies at Duke University showed that a person quick to anger may be quicker to die. Hostility can harm the heart as much as smoking or high blood pressure. Dr. Redford B. Williams Jr. told the American Heart Association that hostility, anger, impatience and high ambitions characterize the Type A heart-attack prone personality. *Half the American population is considered Type A personalities!* They are twice as likely to die of heart disease as Type B people, who are more relaxed and willing to take life as it comes. So if you want to double your chances of living free from heart disease, you must not only watch diet but life-style and emotions! We have to forgive or perish!

Humor and Health: We will here quote the Bible again, "A merry heart doeth good like a medicine." (Prov. 17:22). Medical researchers have discovered that when you laugh, you exercise your heart, lungs, and adrenal glands. You also breathe more deeply, increasing the body's oxygen flow! Dr. Frederic C. McDuffie of the Arthritis Foundation discovered that laughter stimulates the brain to produce endorphins which are hormones that ease pain. "Laughter also makes you feel better by relieving tension." No wonder Amish enjoy laughing!

Insomnia: If you find it hard to sleep at night, try these: 1. Drink camomile tea and eat a lettuce sandwich before retiring. 2. Move to a quieter neighborhood; 3. Simplify your life style (sell off some cars and gadgets!).

Massage: It is a fact that so many people are up tight because of a feeling a alienation from others, as well as too much stress. Amish enjoy having a massage; try foot massage, scalp massage, back massage. There are people dedicated to this ministry of laying on of hands to relieve pain and tension. If you want to keep your ticker ticking, don't wind it too tight!

Modesty: One of the outstanding characteristics of the Amish is their plain dress. They do this for reasons of Biblical modesty, as well as uniformity, and simplicity. The Bible teaches "Women adorn themselves in **modest** apparel, with shamefacedness and sobriety; not with broided hair, or gold, or pearls, or costly array: but...with good works." (I Tim. 2:9-10). "Whose adorning let it not be that outward adorning of plaiting the hair, and of wearing of gold, or of putting on of apparel; but let it be the hidden man of the heart, in that which is not corruptible, **even the ornament of**

a meek and quiet spirit, which is in the sight of God of great price." (IPeter 3:3-4). "If the woman be not covered, let her also be shorn." (I Cor., 11:6). Outward plainness is to allow inward beauty to develop, otherwise one acts a part with cosmetics and costumes.

Prayer and praise: The Bible is full of descriptions of God's people as a people for His praise. "But ye are a chosen generation, . . . that ye should shew forth the praises of Him Who hath called you out of darkness into His marvellous light." (I Peter 2:9). I have never met a *thankful* person who was unhappy. So many people major in criticism, complaining and accusations. God's people major in praise, thanksgiving, encouragement! A spiritually minded Amish person is one who is bubbling over with thanksgiving and praise.

Shunning evil: The Bible admonishes us to shun such things as witchcraft and sorcery, drugs and addiction, drunkenness, gluttony, adultery, malice, fighting, etc. Unruly and rebellious people are to be avoided, just as the devil is to be resisted. We are not only to avoid putting ourselves in situations of temptation but also to avoid all appearance of evil. The strongest sanction of Amish society is placed on avoidance of evil. Furthermore, *evil* should be rebuked. *But the best of us always needs God's forgiveness!*

88

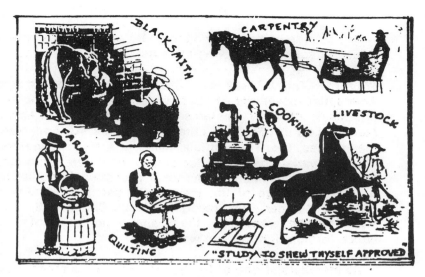

Chapter 9: *Health Hints from the Amish Life Style*

Amish folk remedies are part and parcel of a larger worldwide folk culture. The country people of the world developed a close study of common remedies over the centuries. Some of these remedies were superstitious and some were pragmatic. Let the modern reader beware of too gullibly believing in all folk remedies. On the other hand, let him beware not to become so skeptical that he ignores this area of knowledge. Kipling sympathetically wrote:

> "Excellent herbs had our fathers of old,
> Excellent herbs to ease their pain:
> Alexanders and Marigold,
> Eyebright, Orris and Elecampane,
> Basil, Rocket, Valerian and Rue
> (Almost singing themselves they run),
> Vervain, Dittany, Call-me-to-you,
> Cowslip, Meliot, Rose of the Sun,
> Anything green that grew out of the mould
> *Was an excellent herb to our fathers of old."*

Besides the herbal knowledge. there are other exemplary Amish adaptations to living more healthfully.

Why the Amish Seek to Live Simply: Arising in the Anabaptist movement of 1525. which was a return to the principles of New Testament Christianity, the Amish branched off in 1693 from other Mennonites. All Amish are Mennonites, too. Their official name is Amish Mennonite. There are variations of practice among the different groups. But most emphasize that one must become a Christian by an inward change of life (new birth) before becoming a baptized member. They recognize Jesus Christ as Saviour and Lord. They want to live the Gospel of nonresistant love, which forbids fighting and warfare.

As members of one of the historic Peace Churches, how did the Amish develop into such a nonconformist life-style? From the beginning, together with other **Anabaptists**, they emphasized a holy and devout life. This included simplicity in dress, possessions and work. Coming to the American colonies in the 1740's, the Amish adapted well to the simplicity of pioneer life. They have ever since idealized pioneer simplicity. While other Americans gladly adopted electricity, telephones, radio, television and automobiles, most Amish said these things are unnecessary. They do not want to become slaves of the machine. So they adhere to a simpler lifestyle.

There are some Amish groups, the Beachy Amish Mennonites for example, who do use cars and trucks and electricity and telephones but refuse radio and television. They draw the line at machines of communication which they cannot control, such as TV pumping its pornography and violence into the homes. The strictest Amish are called Old Order Amish Mennonites. All the Amish together probably number less than 100,000.

They live in the U.S. and Canada, Mexico, Salvador, Belize, Honduras, Costa Rica and Paraguay. The Beachy

Amish Mennonites are active in mission outreach in different places and do accept converts from the outside world. But to enter the Old Order Amish, an outsider must convert ot the German language as well as the rest of Amish culture. (The Beachy use English.)

At the end of this chapter, we shall show you a book written by more than 40 converts to the Amish Mennonite faith. It is entitled *Christian and Plain* and is available to anybody who wants to know "how to do it!" We shall also mention other good books which will help you to adapt good things from the Amish culture to your own needs. For example, there is a catalog available of 86 pages of non-electric appliances usable by anybody who wants to simplify his lifestyle. That will also be listed by the end of this chapter.

The Amish in colonial America: As we mentioned, the first Amish settlers arrived in America in the early 1740's. There is also a book available which describes their first settlements and adventures on the frontier. It is entitled "Contentment: The Life and Times of Jacob Hertzler, Pioneer Amish Bishop." It is also listed at the end of this chapter for your further reference. We are introducing you to these books because many have written to us asking for more information.

The Amish pioneer settlers were from the start somewhat different from other pioneers. They would not fight the Indians, for example. They insisted on buying their land rather than expropriating it. They refused to participate in politics or warfare, because their main desire was to build the kingdom of God. Eugene McCarthy once said: "Being in politics is like being a football coach. You have to be smart enough to understand the game and dumb enough to think it's important." The Amish just do not think the whole game plan in politics is their calling. They have the confidence that God will set up the rulers He thinks a country deserves, without their participation except in prayer.

What good are they? So if the Amish do not participate in politics and will not fight in wars, what good are they to any country? They believe that any country rises or falls depending on the presence in it of a righteous remnant of people serious with God. This they believe is their vocation. So they feel it is not the number of atomic bombs, ballistic missiles or armed men that protect a nation, but the number of saints praying for that country!

To most people, this approach is too passive. Are the Amish not **active** in any way to better society? Sure, they raise food, breed better livestock, build solid houses, and besides during times and places of disaster, they will send teams of volunteers to clean up, rebuild, and restore, after floods, fires, earthquakes, and storms. Many communities in the U.S. have been astonished to suddenly see groups of bearded men drive up in busses and vans and begin to clean up and rebuild after some disaster. Who are they? —Amish and Mennonites, helping their stricken neighbors without charge. This service is called M.D.S. or Mennonite Disaster Service.

Furthermore, during wartime, Amish serve in many kinds of alternative civilian service in hospitals, schools, forests. working without wages or for minimal pay, at anything of national benefit instead of military service.

So they are not parasites on society. They have made a contribution. But they just will not walk in step with everybody else and America's freedoms are big enough to allow them to live by their conscience.

What can we learn from them? The whole purpose of this book has been to share with you some of the Amish folk remedies for first aid and survival. Now, here is the address of a genuine Amish herbalist, from whom you can get price lists of all kinds of remedies used by the Amish: **S. Chupp's Herbs & Vitamins,** Herbs Dept. 27539 Londick, Burr Oak, Mich. 49030-9746. Be sure and send a SASE (self-addressed stamped envelope). He ships parcels coast to coast usually by UPS and Air Parcel to Canada and foreign countries. He carries common and rare herbs in stock, even exotic herbs from South America and the Orient. You can ask for his catalog; a donation would be appreciated for postage. It weighs 4 oz. He also has a Saliva Test, Self-awareness Test (SAF), and Hair Analysis Test that his customers take and get good results following his program. But, of course, he cannot diagnose nor prescribe, so don't ask for that.

Would you like help in organizing your own private school? There is an Amish organization called Basic Christian Education, P.O. Box D, Nottawa, Michigan 49075, which will be happy to advise you on how to set up a good, sound curriculum and administer it. They train the teachers and sell the text books, too. Write to them and ask Abe Schwartz *how to do it!* They also help people set up home schooling.

Are you interested in a simpler life, going back to the land? Well, there are hundreds of practical devices listed in the*"Non-electric Good Neighbor Heritage Catalog,"* with 86 large pages for $4.20 postpaid from S. Chupp's Herbs & Vitamins—Book Dept., 27539 Londick, Burr Oak, Michigan 49030-9746. In this catalog you will see listed and priced such practical aids to simple living as wood and coal stoves, grist mills, gasoline or kerosene lamps, refrigerators and freezers run by kerosene, manual washing machines, fruit presses and juicers, food dryers, food mills, hydraulic rams for water power by gravity, wind mills, noodle makers, tools, fly traps, barrels, kegs, treadle sewing machines, farm bess, cheese making equipment, push mowers, etc.!

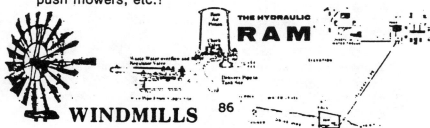

THE HYDRAULIC

RAM

WINDMILLS 86

The Secret of Amish Persistence: Maybe you have wondered why, in the melting pot of America, these Plain People have persisted unassimilated through the centuries? As early as 1797, Isaac Weld Jr. commented on the difference between these Plain People and the average American: "The Germans are fond of settling near each other. When the young men of a family are grown up, they generally endeavor to get a piece of land in the neighborhood of their relations, and by their industry soon make it valuable. The American, on the contrary, is of a roving disposition, is always moving somewheres else, prowling around, buying a place, then moving again. *Restless and discontented with what they possess, they are forever changing.*"

Benjamin Rush in 1789 wrote: "A German farm may be distinguished from the farms of the other citizens of the state by the superior size of their barns. the plain but compact form of their houses, the height of their inclosures, the extent of their orchards, the fertility of their fields, the luxuriance of their meadows, and a general apearance of plenty and neatness in everything that belonged to them."

They never were *superman* but these Plain People always wanted to bring order out of chaos, productivity and fruitfulness out of a wilderness. They fixed on *stability and contentment* instead of *mobility and restlessness.*

Walter M. Kollmorgan in 1942 published a study of the Pennsylvania German farmer, in which he wrote: "The Germans settled on land to *remain there.* They usually lived in compact groups and formed close socioreligious and even economic units. Children could rely on substantial aid from the community as well as from their parents in getting established on farms of their own. *There was much exchange of work* (mutual aid, loans without interest, barn raisings, work bees and "frolics"). *Stability and group settlement were not so general a characteristic of the English-speaking farmers.*"

94

Dr. Benjamin Rush, signer of the Declaration of Independence, after the smoke and fire of the Revolutionary War had cleared, made this wistful comment on the value system of the Plain People: *"Perhaps those German sects of Christians who refuse to bear arms for the shedding of human blood may be preserved by Divine Providence as the center of a circle which shall gradually embrace all nations of the earth in a perpetual treaty of friendship and peace."*

And that, dear reader, is why we are living in this lifestyle! Here are two more books that explain what you want to know:

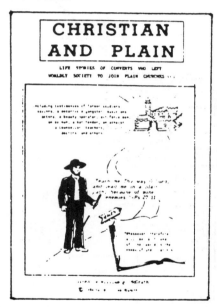

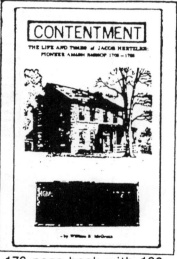

92 page book giving the personal testimonies of 40 men and women who came out of the world to become members of Amish churches. $3.95 postpaid.

176 page book with 130 pictures and drawings about pioneer Amish life in colonial times. $6.95 postpaid.

Order from *S. Chupp's Herbs & Vitamins, Book Dept. 27539 Londick, Burr Oak, Mich. 49030-9746.*

FOOD COMBINING CHART FOR EASIEST DIGESTION

One food at a meal is the most ideal for the easiest and best digestion. Combination of several foods at a meal should be according to the chart below. A meal should not consist of more than four foods.

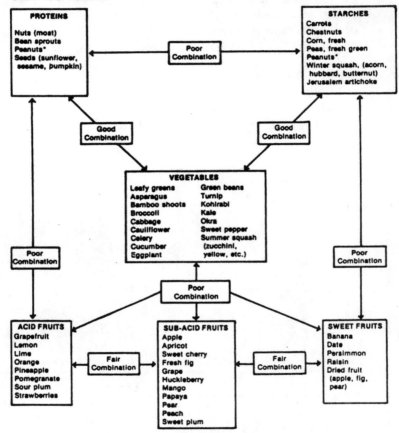

PROTEINS

Nuts (most)
Bean sprouts
Peanuts*
Seeds (sunflower, sesame, pumpkin)

STARCHES

Carrots
Chestnuts
Corn, fresh
Peas, fresh green
Peanuts*
Winter squash, (acorn, hubbard, butternut)
Jerusalem artichoke

Poor Combination

Good Combination

Good Combination

VEGETABLES

Leafy greens
Asparagus
Bamboo shoots
Broccoli
Cabbage
Cauliflower
Celery
Cucumber
Eggplant

Green beans
Turnip
Kohlrabi
Kale
Okra
Sweet pepper
Summer squash (zucchini, yellow, etc.)

Poor Combination

Poor Combination

Poor Combination

ACID FRUITS

Grapefruit
Lemon
Lime
Orange
Pineapple
Pomegranate
Sour plum
Strawberries

Fair Combination

SUB-ACID FRUITS

Apple
Apricot
Sweet cherry
Fresh fig
Grape
Huckleberry
Mango
Papaya
Pear
Peach
Sweet plum

Fair Combination

SWEET FRUITS

Banana
Date
Persimmon
Raisin
Dried fruit (apple, fig, pear)

Avocados, rich in fat, are best combined with green vegetables.
Tomatoes may be best eaten with non-starchy vegetables and proteins.
Melons (all kinds) should be eaten alone.
*Peanuts are considered as protein and starch combinations.

Reprint permission by T. C. Fry

96

AMISH FOLK REMEDIES
by William McGrath

A best seller, explaining Amish Traditions, their proven Herbal Formulas used for generations to stay healthy, happy and stay youthful. Most formulas are available in Herb Gardens or Health Stores. Makes a nice Gift! 104 pages.

Retail $6.99

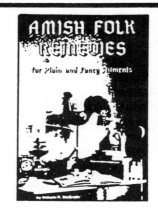

AMERICAN INDIAN FOLK REMEDIES
by William McGrath

Covers Herbs used by the Indians including Pau d'Arco Tea used by many for the incurables! Tells of teas used to overcome impotence, prostate, weight problems, arthritis and much more! 64 pages tells about 50 Indian Herbs, 40 Desert Herbs and 40 Forest Herbs. Pau d'Arco testimonials with book order on request. Retail $6.99

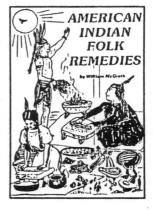

GOD GIVEN HERBS
by William McGrath

New printing - 1986 - 96 pages. First distributor ordered 500 books! Ailments from Arthritis, cancer to whooping cough. Remedies given. This Book tells on pages 33 & 34 how he was cured from crippling rheumatoid arthritis, using simple homeopathic remedies! What the Bible says about sickness and health, page 6. Live foods that work as Herbal Medicines. Retail $6.99

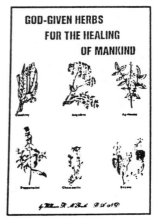

Purchase all three books
for $19.95 + 1.50 P&H

Index

100

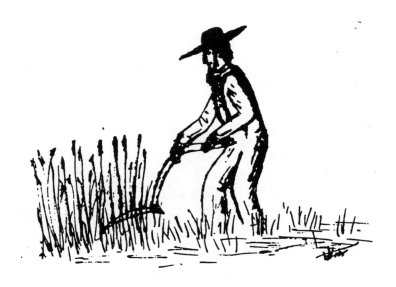

Notes